PROBIOTICS FOR
LIFE

PROBIOTICS FOR LIFE

A HEALTHY AND ENERGETIC LIFE

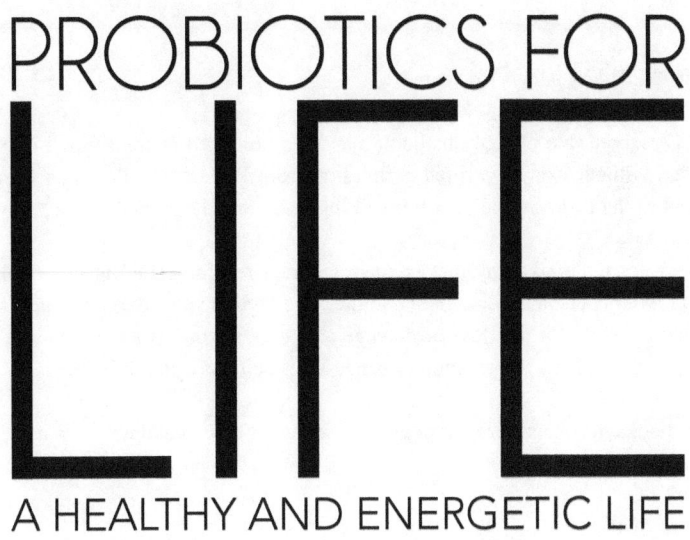

Your Guide to Understanding How Probiotics
and Their Functions Benefit Your Body

ALBERT BRECKER

iUniverse LLC
Bloomington

PROBIOTICS FOR LIFE
A Healthy and Energetic Life

iUniverse books may be ordered through booksellers or by contacting:

iUniverse LLC
1663 Liberty Drive
Bloomington, IN 47403
www.iuniverse.com
1-800-Authors (1-800-288-4677)

ISBN: 978-1-4759-9426-1 (sc)
ISBN: 978-1-4759-9427-8 (hc)
ISBN: 978-1-4759-9428-5 (e)

Printed in the United States of America

iUniverse rev. date: 03/17/2014

*Learn how probiotics enhance
and strengthen your digestive
and immune systems for a healthier life.*

CONTENTS

PREFACE

My introduction to the world of probiotics came totally by surprise.

By accident, I stumbled upon an amazing probiotic supplement formula that saved my feet from years of terrible fungal infections, otherwise known as athlete's foot.

I am certainly no serious athlete, but I have suffered from athlete's foot fungus for years—really bad athlete's foot. My feet were on fire, and the skin of my toes and feet was constantly itching and peeling. I was even hospitalized with cellulitis, a serious skin disease related to the athlete's foot fungus.

As a regimen for overall intestinal and digestive well-being, my health-care professionals recommended consuming good probiotic supplements. Since some probiotics perform better than others do, I experimented with different probiotic formulas. The reasons were completely unrelated to my athlete's foot problems.

Unknowingly, I hit upon an amazing formula, and I suddenly discovered that my nagging foot fungus began to clear up. It took a couple of short weeks—and it didn't return as long as I kept taking the supplements!

I offered this incredulous formula to many friends who suffered from the same foot skin fungus. They too were surprised that their skin fungus cleared up.

There has not been any manufacturer of probiotics so far that has claimed that its probiotics could battle athlete's foot.

I knew I had discovered something big.

If a formula is so powerful that it can clear up outer skin fungus, imagine how much fungus it must eliminate inside the body.

I began a ten-year journey of researching and studying the benefits and effects of probiotics on the human body. I consulted with many prominent microbiologists, chemists, and health professionals specializing in the field of probiotic nutrition. I learned about strong, potent formulas of probiotics that could benefit the entire human body from head to toe—literally from dandruff to athlete's foot.

After researching and experimenting various potent and effective formulas, I discovered formulas that have the amazing potential of relieving and soothing a myriad of maladies. These range from athlete's foot fungus to cramps of colicky infants and from dandruff to the flu. It also could improve LDL cholesterol, constipation, indigestion, IBS, colitis, and Crohn's disease. It could eliminate yeast infections and much more.

The culmination of ten years of scientific research is inculcated in this book, which espouses the attributes of probiotics.

> In *Probiotics for Life* I will take you on a journey through the largely uncharted waters and relatively unknown new world of probiotics.
>
> You will learn how to strengthen your immune system, cleanse your digestive system, live healthier, and live longer. You will also understand how probiotics offer a host of benefits for the entire immune system, digestive system, and many vital organs of the whole human body.

We are just at the beginning of major discoveries in the field of probiotics.

Albert Brecker
President and founder of ProDermix Institute of Probiotics
President of American Nutrition Consultants,
authorized distributors of ProDermix®

INTRODUCTION

Probiotics have been with us since the creation of mankind. The discovery of the benefits and functions of probiotics is the fruit of research by Dr. Elie Metchnikoff at the Pasteur Institute in 1908. The universal understanding of the need and accomplishments of probiotics began some thirty years ago. New discoveries and revelations of the power and success of probiotics in human health and well-being are now being understood and proliferated by the probiotic manufacturing community.

The science of probiotics is yet to be understood and accepted universally in the world of medicine. Even the world of fans of alternative health solutions has not yet fully grasped the phenomenal potential health benefits that probiotics have to offer.

The European community is heavily involved in probiotic research, notably such countries as France, Italy, Germany, Norway, Finland, and Switzerland, among others. In the United States, probiotics are still on the "back burner" regarding research and marketing.

Dr. Mary Ellen Sanders, chairperson of CAST (Council for Agricultural Science and Technology)[1] task force, published an in-depth report on probiotics titled *Probiotics: Their Potential to Impact Human Health*. She states that, as I paraphrase her words, the list of benefits from probiotics seems too diverse to be possible to the average layperson. Once one realizes that probiotics have the ability to positively impact and colonize any region of the body locally and systemically, only then will the wide range of benefits be appreciated.

---

[1]   CAST is an organization that lobbies Congress on the health and nutrition of meat and agricultural products.

We are presently sitting on a vast, untapped reservoir of health-related resources and benefits in the world of probiotics that has yet to be discovered. New and exciting areas of potential benefits are being discovered constantly in the field of probiotics.

The wide ranges of benefits cover a broad spectrum of areas of successful internal and external body health. The multiple benefits range from the effective soothing of atopic dermatitis in infants to anticarcinogenic activity in the colon, and from the elimination of cradle cap in infants to the defeat of athlete's foot fungus in adults. These and many more are only some of the new revelations and discoveries that are being discovered in the arena of probiotic research day after day. The steady stream of new findings is genuinely awesome!

At the summary of this report, more than fifty attributes of probiotics are identified for the overall health of the entire body. The list goes from athlete's foot improvement to colicky infant soothing, and from LDL cholesterol improvement to yeast infection relief and much more. We have a long road of exciting discoveries ahead.

Sales of probiotics in the United States in the year 2000 were below $450 million. In 2010, sales topped $1.1 billion. This figure includes sales of probiotic supplements and sales of probiotic ingredients used in foods like yogurt.[2] European Union countries and Asian countries are far more advanced in their research, knowledge, and consumption of probiotics than the Americans are. Their sales are climbing quickly too.

The awareness of the benefits of probiotics and the dissemination of that knowledge is still in its infancy. To wit, as of the year 2007, Microsoft Word 2007 did not have the word *probiotic* in its spell-check dictionary.

---

[2]   lEN/US sales of probiotics/8594.

CHAPTER ONE

Discovery of Probiotics!

Old-World Probiotics

Probiotics are the supplemental form of healthy bacteria that inhabit your gastrointestinal tract. These healthy flora (friendly bacteria) are essential for the health and proper functioning of the organs of the body in general, and the digestive tract in particular.

Before the advent of modern science and medicine, a prime source of healthy bacteria for the well-being of the intestinal tract was fermented borscht and sauerkraut.

Your grandmothers used to make homemade sour borscht from beets. The beets were soaked in barrels of water and stored in a warm environment. Towels and blankets were wrapped around the barrels to keep them warm until the beets fermented. In approximately four to six weeks, they produced a thick lather of fermentation.

The fermentation was the healthy bacteria of flora, which is now known as probiotics. The scientific names of the healthy flora are Lactobacillus acidophilus and Lactobacillus bulgaricus. These live bacteria organisms are now included in yogurt and aid in digesting foods and strengthening the immune system.

The actual recipe for real homemade sour borscht is Grandma's best kept secret.

A laboratory test was performed where live E. coli bacteria was placed on top of the healthy bacterial fermentation of homemade sour borscht (live probiotics), and within a short period the E. coli bacteria was totally consumed or destroyed by the fermentation (or probiotics). E. coli, salmonella, shigella, and many other pathogens are among the unhealthy bacteria that are destroyed by probiotics.

Bottled borscht sold in supermarkets today is a distant imitation of the real thing and has a very scant positive effect on your health.

The healthy attributes of sour fermented borscht are already mentioned in the Talmud as of 1,800 years ago. The Talmud discusses various foods that are beneficial for different organs in the human body.

Caraway seeds, for example, are mentioned as being extremely beneficial for vascular health.[3] However, they have a damaging effect on one's eyesight.[4]

Conversely, there are foods that are good for the eyes but are detrimental to the heart and vascular system.

Sour borscht, which is fermented naturally from beets, is presented by the Talmud as beneficial for the eyes and the vascular system simultaneously. The Talmud further mentions that borscht also kills bad bacteria in the digestive system.[5] Borscht is perhaps one of the precursors of modern-day probiotics. It was already identified close to two thousand years ago as the media of healthy flora for many vital organs of the human body.

A wise old man who lived in South Brooklyn used to research nutritional benefits for longevity of life. He would extol the benefits of caraway soup for vascular health and well-being. He perfected his own homemade recipe for caraway soup. He would constantly urge his friends to eat caraway soup for a healthy heart and long life. He lived to a healthy and ripe age of ninety years. However, for the last twelve years of his life he wore eyeglasses with lenses as thick as

---

[3]   Tractate Eruvin 29A.

[4]   Tractate Pesachim 42B, Rashi's commentary.

[5]   Tractate Brachot 40A.

magnifying glasses. Obviously, his heart may have functioned well, but the caraway soup took its toll on his eyes.

Perhaps, had he known that fermented borscht can deliver "the best of both worlds," a healthy heart and healthy eyes, he would have extolled the benefits of borscht instead.

Sauerkraut is another natural medium for healthy probiotics for the digestive system. Fermented sauerkraut has similar properties to sour borscht and is very healthy for the digestive tract. Fresh cabbage is populated with healthy bacteria that are released upon proper fermentation conditions. *Kraut* is "cabbage" in German, thus sauerkraut is sour or fermented cabbage.

Increased awareness and popularity of the functions of probiotics are reawakening interest in the age-old leafy vegetable cabbage in its spiced and fermented stage that is known as sauerkraut. As the awareness of probiotics continues to be expounded, sour borscht and sauerkraut would probably be elevated to celebrity status in the natural and health food industry.

LET OUR JOURNEY BEGIN!
Ship ahoy!

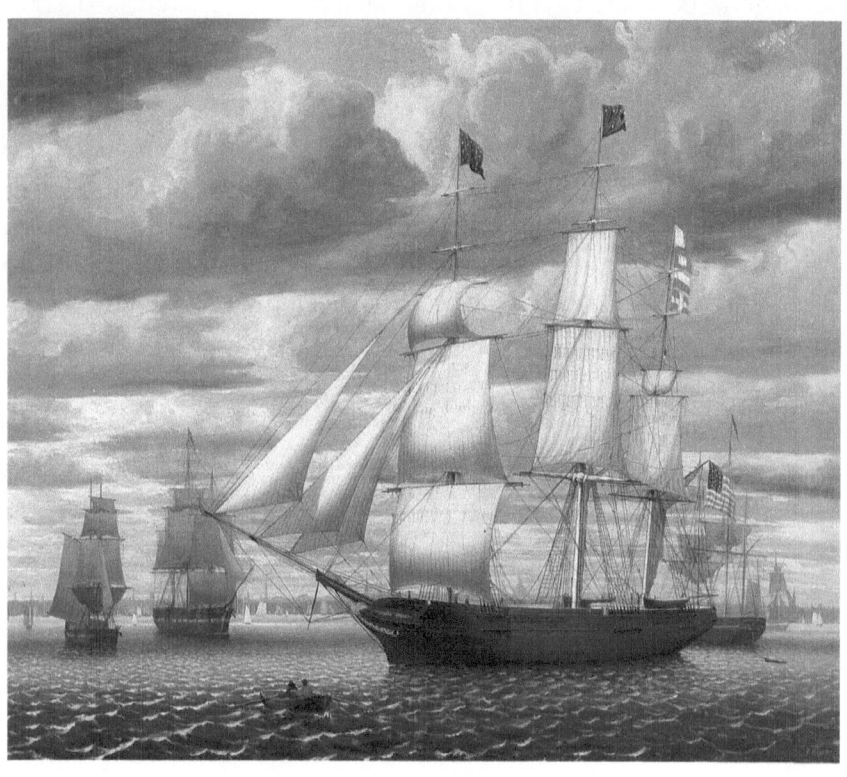

Probiotics Assist the Royal Navy in 1758

Spain, Portugal, Holland, and Great Britain were competing for world dominance of the spice trade centered on the Far East, particularly in East Indies (Indonesia). Trading in spices was very lucrative in the 1700s and brought great wealth to the countries.

While Spain, Portugal, and Holland were angling to outdo each other in naval supremacy, Great Britain was quietly building its navy into a supreme, world-class navy.

In that era, sailors at sea endured extreme hardships that made it physically difficult to remain seaborne for a lengthy period of time. Malnutrition, seaborne sicknesses, and many other ailments claimed the lives of *more than* 50 percent of the sailors on most voyages. They lacked refrigeration, and their fresh food supply depleted and spoiled in very short time. Scurvy and other debilitating diseases plagued many seafarers.

Magellan lost 80 percent of his crew while crossing the Pacific Ocean. Commodore George Anson was commissioned to lead a squadron of British ships in the Pacific in the 1740s to raid Spanish shipping. He lost thirteen hundred of his original two thousand crew members.[6]

Captain James Cook was commissioned by the Royal Navy in 1758 to explore a new route for the spice trade and take possession of new territories for the Crown. In order to succeed, a system had to be established whereas sailors could endure long, hardy voyages. He successfully implemented many hygienic procedures at sea.

He was aware of the importance of specific foods needed to ward off sickness and strengthen the body's immune system. Special fruits and foods that supplied effective vitamins and probiotics were stored onboard to assure the health and strength of the sailors.

---

[6]   Jonathan Lamb, "Captain Cook and the Scourge of Scurvy," BBC, last modified February 17, 2011, http://www.bbc.co.uk/history/british/empire_seapower/captaincook_scurvy_01.shtml.

He identified sauerkraut as an important source for strengthening the health of his sailors. It became a staple food for his sailors. Sauerkraut is fermented cabbage, which contains an abundance of super-healthy flora (probiotics) that support the immune system and cleanse the digestive tract of the body. It also helps to ward off intestinal digestive diseases. It eases constipation and soothes sufferers of diarrhea.

He also discovered that the scurvy disease was due to insufficient intake of ascorbic acid (vitamin C). His ships always carried an ample supply of lemon juice and other citrus fruits.

Thanks to Captain Cook's in-depth knowledge of proper diet and hygiene, 90 percent of his sailors survived the lengthy voyages of his expeditions.[7] The scourge of scurvy was completely eliminated from the Royal Navy by the end of the eighteenth century.

Hence, probiotics played a major role in the many successful expeditions of Captain Cook and the Royal British Navy. (The term *probiotics* was coined two centuries later.)

The Modern-Day Discovery of Probiotics

At the turn of the twentieth century, Dr. Elie Metchnikoff, a Nobel Laureate biologist, discovered the benefits of Lactobacillus acidophilus and bulgaricus.[8] While studying the "laws governing the duration of human life" at the Pasteur Institute in Paris, Dr. Metchnikoff concluded that a person could achieve a life span of ninety to one hundred years.

The *New York Times* of January 18, 1908, ran a headline page article entitled "The Prolongation of Life," regarding the achievements and discoveries of Dr. Metchnikoff relating to his studies and recommendations of a healthy lifestyle for people.

---

[7]   Ibid.
[8]   Metchnikoff, *The Prolongation of Life* (London: G.P. Putnam's Sons, 1907).

He studied people in Bulgaria (hence the name bulgaricus) and surrounding states who lived healthy lives up to 114 years of age. Most of the elderly who reached that age were physically and mentally active. He attributed their longevity and general good state of health to their consuming of healthy sour milk and buttermilk. The healthy ingredients therein are now called Lactobacillus acidophilus and Lactobacillus bulgaricus and are classified as probiotics.

The *New York Times* elaborates about the remarkable longevity of life that Dr. Metchnikoff attributes to the "vegetable kingdom." Probiotics are manufactured from various dairy media, including sour milk, and several vegetation media, including soybeans, cabbage, beets, etc. Today, there are lactose-free probiotics and soy-free probiotics for persons intolerant to those media. Dr. Metchnikoff's studies were more far-reaching and elaborate than acidophilus and probiotics. Nevertheless, he is known as the father of modern probiotics.

The actual term *probiotics* was coined by the researchers Lilly and Stilwell in their studies in 1965.[9] In 1989, a study entitled, "Probiotics in Man and Animals," from a researcher by the name of Fuller, popularized the term probiotics.[10]

Probiotics are becoming ever more important to health-care practitioners and medical doctors as their properties and functions of relieving the digestive system are witnessed daily. But it is not only the digestive system that benefits from probiotics. The entire immune system is enhanced with probiotic intake. Thanks to probiotics, the epidermis of the human body enjoys improvement from many fungal conditions, including but not limited to athlete's foot fungus, dandruff, candida, and some forms of eczema.

---

[9]   Lilly and Stilwell, "Probiotics: Growth-Promoting Factors, Etc.," 1965.
[10] R. Fuller, "Probiotics in Man and Animals," 1989.

The Gift of Probiotics to Our Generation

The Generation Gap

Generations ago, people consumed wholesome foods, with plenty of legumes and protein. Necessary vitamins, minerals, and digestive enzymes present in the food were directly digested and absorbed into the GI tract and distributed to the vital organs systematically. There wasn't much need for probiotic supplements to aid digestion and absorption of vital nutrients into the human body.

Additionally, probiotic-producing foods were regularly consumed as part of their natural menu. Unpasteurized sour milk, buttermilk, and yogurt were part of their daily diet. Sauerkraut, cabbage, beets, borscht, and other probiotic-producing legumes were part of everyday meals. People consumed natural probiotics constantly.

Now one might ponder this question: How serious and truthful could this probiotic idea be regarding longevity of life ("prolongation of life")?[11] If the former generations lived a healthier lifestyle and were stronger due to their consumption of healthier foods and flora, why was their average lifespan much shorter than ours today?

The answer is logical and very clear.

People of previous generations led a stronger and healthier life on a day-to-day basis. Their bodies were stronger, and their lifestyle was wholesome. Although their average life span was considerably shorter than today, the quality of life was more energetic and healthier.

However, the prime reason most people did not live to a ripe old age was due to the poor hygienic environment and the rampant plagues resulting from their unhealthy living conditions.

---

[11] Metchnikoff, *The Prolongation of Life*.

Many worldwide ailments and illnesses, such as the bubonic plague, the black death, cholera, and dysentery, among others, spread rapidly and wiped out entire cities and states because they lacked proper hygiene.

In the late 1800s, Dr. Joseph Lister discovered why the majority of postsurgery patients died after their successful surgery.[12] He discovered that the patients died from infections transmitted from one patient to the next. The surgeons were not aware of proper antiseptic procedures and did not cleanse themselves properly between one procedure and the next. The surgeons themselves were the carriers of the bacteria from patient to patient.

Dr. Joseph Lister implemented a simple basic rule that physicians adhere to until this day, requiring all doctors to wash their hands and cleanse properly between one patient and the next. This basic hygienic philosophy led the medical establishment to implement proper hygiene in all hospitals and medical procedures. Millions of lives have been saved as a result.

Prior to Dr. Lister's discovery, the medical community lacked basic knowledge regarding treatment of external and internal infections. That took a major toll of lives during war and peacetime. Soldiers wounded on the battlefield died mostly from their infected wounds rather than the gravity of the wound itself.

Years later with the advent of the wonder drug penicillin,[13] most troops on the war front survived their initial wound infections. The penicillin drug conquered many difficult inner and outer infections. It indeed contributed to a longer and healthier life in developed countries.

---

[12]   "Joseph Lister," Wikipedia, last modified March 20, 2013, http://en.wikipedia.org/wiki/Joseph_Lister,_1st_Baron_Lister.

[13]   Alexander Fleming discovered penicillin in 1928. "Penicillin," Wikipedia, last modified March 24, 2013, http://en.wikipedia.org/wiki/Penicillin.

Dr. Elie Metchnikoff came upon his discovery of the "prolongation of life"[14] through probiotics. He studied Bulgarian peasants living long and healthy lives in farming communities. They lived to the ripe age of around one hundred years.

The Bulgarians he studied did not live in central Europe and were far away from major commerce centers where diseases were easily spread from city to city by traveling merchants and tourists. They lived in small towns and villages, farther removed form Europe's main commerce corridor, in basically healthy environments. They consumed healthy foods, and their eating habits consisted of healthy legumes and foods laden with protein and probiotics. Compared to the rest of Europe, the Bulgarian peasants were the exception and did enjoy longevity.

If the European community-at-large had similar pristine living conditions, they probably would have lived much longer as well.

Fast-Forward to Our Generation

Our generation is fortunate to live longer because of our development of sterile hygienic conditions on a personal, daily basis. We are also fortunate to have championed major cures and remedies to halt the spread of rampant diseases and infection.

But our generation lacks the physical and mental energy and stamina of previous generations, due to our poor dietary menus and eating habits. In today's super-unhealthy environment, fast food outlets churn out daily menus laden with hydrogenated fats, heavy starches, and carbohydrates. These types of food strain, abuse and weigh heavily on your digestive system. They tend to destroy the healthy flora (bacteria) adhering to the mucosal lining of the digestive tract that battle destructive pathogens and many other harmful contaminants. Worse, processed soft drinks and sugar-filled pastries cling to your inner intestines and obstruct

---

[14]   Metchnikoff, *The Prolongation of Life.*

the absorption of the healthy enzymes, vitamins, and minerals into the body's organs. A wide array of bacteria, pathogens, and carcinogens are then allowed to invade the gastrointestinal tract, because of unhealthy meal choices and poor eating habits.

Thanks to modern probiotics, a great gift to our generation, there is now a strong and lasting remedy!

Probiotics is the long-awaited solution that is becoming familiar and ever more popular in the area of digestive health and wellness.

Acidophilus, among other probiotics, assists in the growth of new flora in the gut and helps maintain a healthy bacterial balance in the gastrointestinal tract.

More than one hundred trillion units of healthy microbiota inhabit your gastrointestinal tract. The healthy bacteria continuously battle the harmful bacteria. Your digestive tract requires healthy flora to counterbalance the fungal properties propagated by the unfriendly flora.

Growing and multiplying good bacteria in the gut is why people take probiotics. The science has evolved into a major industry and network of labs manufacturing many probiotic strains and blends that aid in the healthy digestion and absorption of necessary nutrients, vitamins, minerals, and digestive enzymes in the gastrointestinal tract and beyond. The medical profession today already recognizes the significance of probiotics as assistance in digestion and absorption of vitamins and minerals in the GI tract and its abilities to enhance the immune system.[15]

---

[15] My Health News Daily, "Probiotics to Ease Gut Problems," November 1, 2011.

CHAPTER TWO

Defining Probiotics!

What Are Probiotics?

The World Health Organization (WHO) defines probiotics as "live microorganisms which when administered in adequate amounts confer a health benefit on the host."

Defining the Term *Probiotic*

Let us first define the term *probiotic*. *Biotic* means life. It usually refers to the life of bacteria, the viral or fungal bacteria that creates sicknesses and maladies. To battle and neutralize those fungal bacteria, the medical and pharmaceutical establishments have researched and developed many different types of *anti*biotics. Nobody wants these bacteria to remain alive. The antibiotics destroy their life.

The term *probiotic* relates to the healthy, friendly bacteria in your digestive tract that you want to multiply in your gastrointestinal tract for the well-being of your health. Everyone wants these friendly bacteria to remain alive and healthy and to multiply, hence the term *probiotic*.

Probiotics are not enzymes, vitamins, or minerals, nor are they chemical compounds.

Natural probiotics are microorganisms that are live in your intestines.

Manufactured probiotics are *controlled bacteria* (i.e., friendly flora, healthy and beneficial bacteria) that are manufactured in controlled laboratory environments. The healthy flora or bacteria called probiotics are grown, fermented, and cultivated from various media, such as dairy, vegetables, beans, beets, and others.

Probiotics work together with and complement the vitamins, minerals, and nutrients the human body needs for its vital functions.

Are Probiotics Different from Vitamins, Minerals, and Enzymes?

Functions of Vitamins, Minerals, Enzymes, and Probiotics

What are the different functions of vitamins, minerals, digestive enzymes, and probiotics?

Vitamins, minerals, and digestive enzymes are essential to the well-being of the human body and its organs.

Vitamins

Vitamins are essential to life; they assist the process of releasing energy from food into the organs of the body, and they regulate metabolism. They work together with the enzymes, enabling the body to absorb and distribute the energy into the system. There are several categories of vitamins; there are fat-soluble vitamins and water-soluble vitamins. Vitamins A, D, E, and K are fat-soluble. If you have a fat-free diet, your body may not absorb these vitamins. The water-soluble vitamins consist of B1, B2, B3, B5, B6, B12, C, and several more. These cannot be stored in the body and must be replenished daily.

Minerals

Minerals are very important for the proper composition of body fluids. Minerals give your body sustained energy. They build and feed the cells of the blood and bones of the entire body.

Some of the more commonly known vital minerals for the body's healthy functioning are magnesium, potassium, iron, and zinc. Other important minerals that your body needs are calcium, sodium, boron, copper, cobalt, chromium, iodine, sulphur, selenium, vanadium, silicon, and phosphorus.

Magnesium is one of the most important minerals that strengthens and energizes thirty-six organs of the human body.[16] Magnesium strengthens the cardiovascular system of your body. Probiotics assist in the absorption process of magnesium and other minerals into your vital organs.

Enzymes

Enzymes are naturally produced in the salivary glands and in the stomach. One of those enzymes is salivary amylase. They comingle with the food and assist in their breaking down to a soluble state in order that the vitamins and minerals are absorbed into the gastrointestinal tract. Additional human-manufactured enzymes are prescribed for consumption when the body does not have the ability to produce enough enzymes to satisfy the digestive system. Commonly used manufactured supplemental enzymes include catalase, peptidase, papain (papaya), and bromelain (pineapple).

---

[16]   Michael and Mary Dan Eades, MD, *Protein Power* (John Wiley & Sons Inc) 2001.

Probiotics

The gastrointestinal tract ("GI") (from the esophagus into the stomach and the intestines to the anus) is a complex micro-ecosystem in which the mucosal lining of the host coexists with trillions of microorganisms that live on or are attached to the lining. Among the microorganisms that inhabit the GI tract are probiotic bacteria, also known as intestinal microbiota, which help maintain the health of the GI tract.

Probiotics support the intestinal microflora against antagonizing microorganisms. Enzymes aid the digestive system. Probiotics assist the GI tract to absorb minerals, vitamins, and other necessary nutrients into the vital organs and support the functions of the immune system.

The gastrointestinal tract has many finger-like protrusions along the intestinal walls. These projections are called villi. Covering the villi are hair-like projections called microvilli. After the food is processed in the stomach with the biles and peptic acids that break down the food particles, those particles enter the intestines and the vitamins and minerals are absorbed into the body's organs through the villi and microvilli. The unhealthy diet of the fast food consumers, such as sugar, carbs, enhanced dairy products, and fat-laden pastries and cakes, create layers of gunk and glue that obstruct the villi from absorbing minerals and vitamins into the body.

The intestinal microbiota reside in the ileum (small intestine) and in the colon (large intestine).

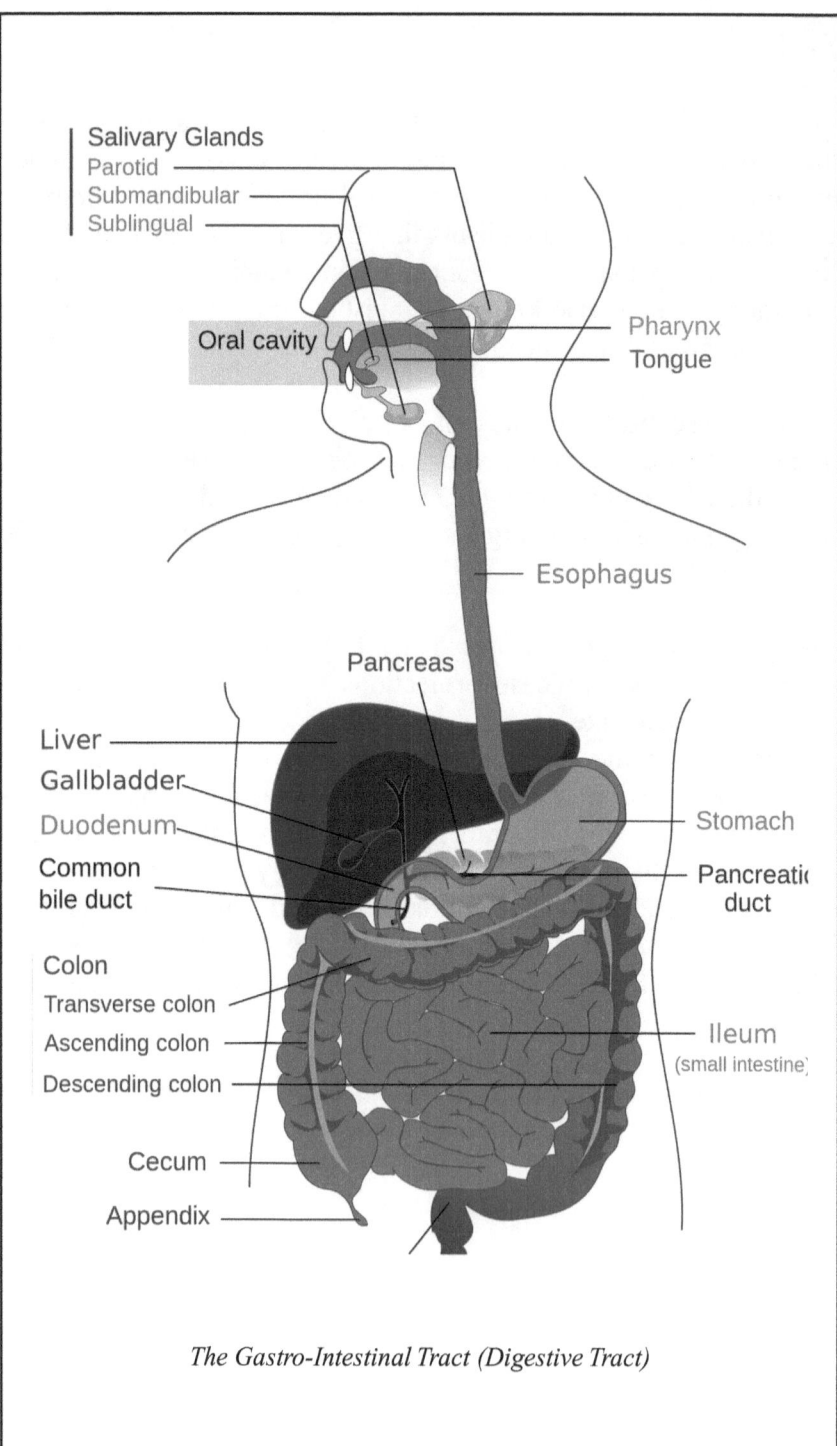

The Gastro-Intestinal Tract (Digestive Tract)

Functions of the Gastrointestinal Tract

The gastrointestinal tract starts at the mouth and continues all the way down until the anus. The GI tract releases hormones to aid in digestion and absorption of important vitamins, minerals, and enzymes.

The GI tract consists of the upper intestinal tract and the lower intestinal tract.

The upper part of the GI tract is the esophagus and the stomach.

The lower intestinal tract consists of the small intestine and the large intestine.

The Small Intestine

Digestive juices from the pancreas and bile from the gallbladder mix in the small intestine to break down proteins and bile and emulsify fats with other enzymes to help neutralize the HCl in the stomach. Parts of the small intestine also have villi that absorb vitamins and minerals into the bloodstream.

The Large Intestine

The large intestine consists of ascending colon, transverse colon, and the descending colon. The main function of the colon is to absorb water and help in the elimination of waste from the body. It also contains beneficial bacteria that produce necessary vitamins for the body.

Immune Function

The stomach has a low pH factor (from 1 to 4) that is fatal for many microorganisms entering it. Also, the mucus of the membranes in the GI tract (containing IgA antibodies) neutralizes many pathogenic microorganisms. Additional enzymes in the GI tract defeat and detoxify harmful bacteria that enter the GI tract. The GI tract is a major part of the body's immune system.

Digestion Timetable

It is estimated by gastrointestinal researchers that the time it takes for food to empty from the stomach into the intestines is approximately four to five hours. Emptying from the small intestine to the large intestine is approximately two to three hours. Finally, transit through the colon takes thirty to forty hours.

Probiotics aid in the digestion and immune response of the GI tract. They also help the digestive juices penetrate smoothly through the small intestine and into the large intestine. This helps to ease the elimination process and relieves symptoms of constipation, thereby speeding the transit time through the colon.

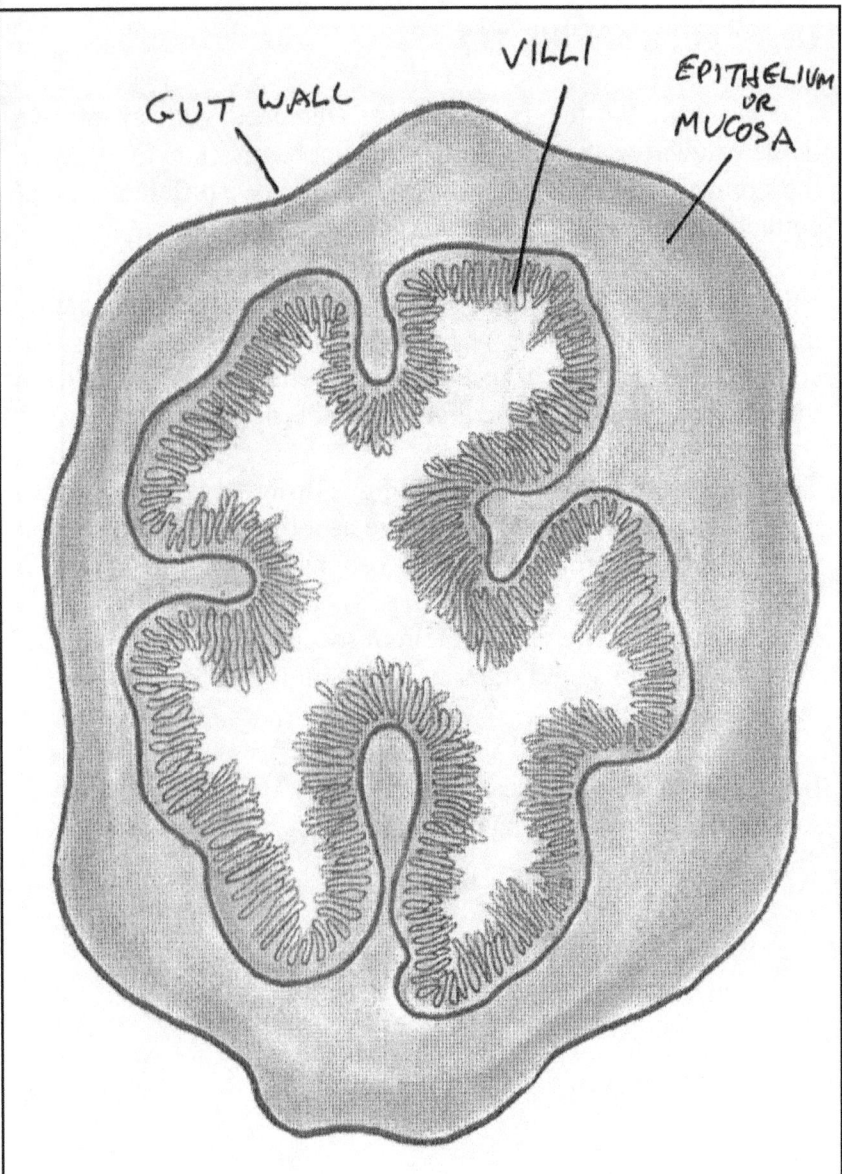

GUT WALL

VILLI

EPITHELIUM
OR
MUCOSA

Healthy (Absorbent) Villi

A healthy GI tract has healthy villi as shown above.

Description of Villi

The gut wall (or the intestinal wall) is lined with absorptive tissue known as "epithelium." The esophagus (the food pipe), the stomach, and the small intestine each have a different type of epithelium lining. (see illustration on page 25)

Villi are the hairlike protrusions from the epithelium coating the inner side of the gut wall. Microvilli are minute hairs that comprise the villi and absorb all the minerals and vitamins from the food traveling down the digestive tract (or GI tract).

The purpose of the epithelium lining is different in each part. In the esophagus it is mostly protective as a lining to guard against foreign objects from damaging the esophageal wall.

In the small intestine, the epithelium specializes in absorption of vitamins, minerals, and other nutrition into the bloodstream and the vital body organs.

In the stomach, it is organized into gastric pits and glands to secrete the necessary enzymes that aid in food breakdown and digestion.

Unhealthy villi do not have the separated tentacles able to absorb and digest the minerals and nutrients of the food. They cling together because of the fatty substances from the unhealthy foods consumed from most fast food diets.

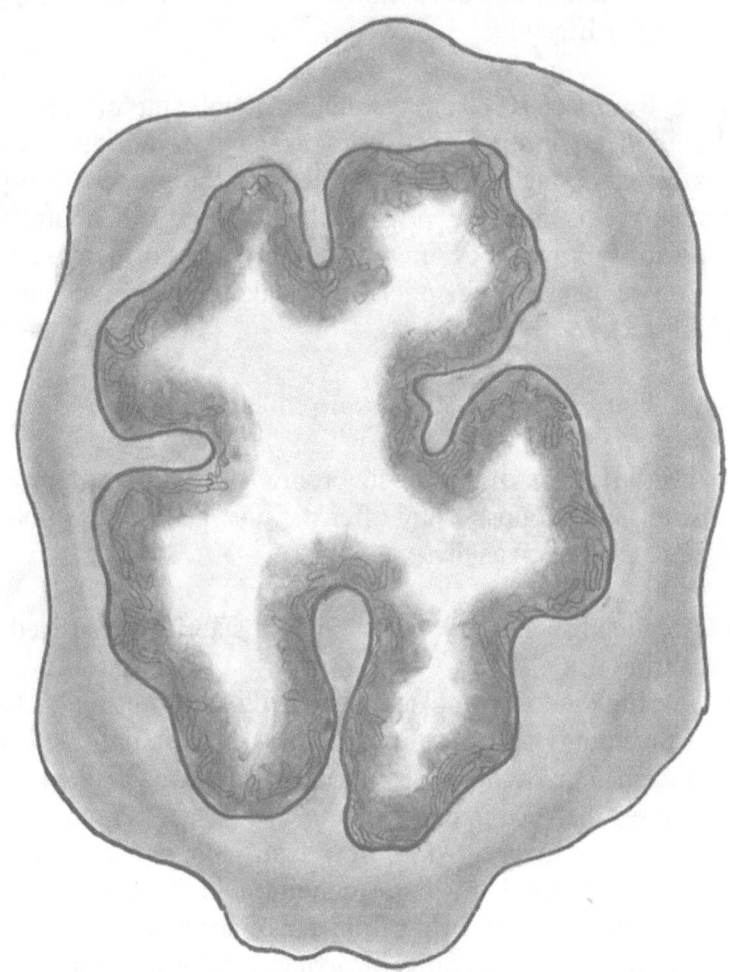

Unhealthy (Clogged) Villi

Probiotics antagonize and battle the mucosal fungus created by pathogenic bacteria that cling to the villi in the intestinal tract and tend to restrict the flow of beneficial nourishment into the system. The cells of healthy flora engulf the pathogenic bacteria and deprive them of their pathogenic and carcinogenic capabilities. Thus, your healthier digestive system promises you more longevity and a healthier lifestyle.

Probiotic live bacteria facilitate the metabolizing of undigested food components in the digestive tract. They also aid the intestinal walls to produce the secretions needed for the proper absorption of vital nutrients into the organs of the body. When probiotics are coupled with prebiotic ingredients, there is an increase in the absorption of magnesium, potassium, calcium, and zinc into the intestinal tract.[17]

Probiotics coupled with prebiotics are called synbiotics.

Within the GI tract of the host, probiotic bacteria are provided with shelter and support. They offer the host a variety of potential therapeutic uses, such as these:

- Replacing healthy intestinal bacteria destroyed by antibiotics
- Aiding digestion and suppressing disease-causing bacteria
- Preventing and treating diarrhea, including infectious diarrhea, particularly from rotavirus (a virus that commonly causes diarrhea in children)
- Treating overgrowth of "bad" organisms in the gastrointestinal tract (a condition that tends to cause diarrhea and may occur from use of antibiotics)
- Alleviating symptoms of irritable bowel syndrome and, possibly, inflammatory bowel disease (such as Crohn's disease and ulcerative colitis)[18]

---

[17] E. Scharrer and T. Lutz, "Effects of Absorption of Magnesium, etc. by the Colon," Z. Ernharungswiss (1990).

[18] Heidi Splete, Internal Medicine News, Feb. 15, 2008 (from Highbeam Research). Studies reported by Dr. Leo Dieleman, University of Alberta,

- Preventing and/or reducing the recurrence of yeast infections, urinary tract infections, and cystitis (bladder inflammation)
- Improving lactose absorption and digestion in people who are lactose intolerant
- Enhancing the immune response

Digestion, Probiotics, and Basic Exercise

Digestion is the mechanical and chemical breakdown of food into smaller components that are more easily absorbed, as into a blood stream, for instance.[19]

When food enters the mouth, digestion starts by the action of mastication, a form of mechanical digestion, and the contact of saliva. Saliva, which is secreted by the salivary glands, contains salivary amylase, an enzyme that starts the digestion of starch in the food. After undergoing mastication and starch digestion, the food will be in the form of a small, round, slurry mass. It will then travel down the esophagus and into the stomach by the action of peristalsis. Gastric juice in the stomach starts protein digestion. The gastric juice mainly contains hydrochloric acid and pepsin. As these two chemicals may damage the stomach wall, mucus is secreted by the stomach, providing a slimy layer that acts as a shield against the damaging effects of the chemicals.

Mechanical mixing occurs by peristalsis, which includes waves of muscular contractions that move along the stomach wall and the entire digestive tract. (See illustration of gut wall.) Basic exercise, such as brisk walking, is very important in order to energize the muscular contractions that transport the food down through the digestive tract. Elderly people often develop digestive problems, mainly due to their lack of exercise.

Edmonton.
[19] Wikipedia/digestion/last modified/MARCH 29/2013.

Peristalsis allows the mass of food to further mix with the digestive enzymes. After some time, typically an hour or two, the resulting thick liquid is called chyme.

When the pyloric sphincter valve opens (where the small intestine [duodenum] and stomach connect), chyme enters the duodenum (the beginning of the small intestine) where it mixes with digestive enzymes from the pancreas and then passes through the small intestine, in which digestion continues. When the chyme is fully digested, it is absorbed into the blood. Ninety-five percent of absorption of nutrients occurs in the small intestine. Some vitamins, such as biotin and vitamin K produced by bacteria in the colon (microflora or probiotics), are also absorbed into the blood in the colon. Waste material is eliminated from the rectum during defecation.[20]

Proper digestion and absorption of food into the intestinal tract are reliant on two important factors. The two factors are exercise and live, active microflora, or probiotics, in the digestive tract.

Peristalsis is the action of muscular contractions that push the food downward throughout the whole gastrointestinal tract, past the large intestine. This is the part that relies on exercise. When one exercises well, the internal organs of the body are stimulated and respond well, doing their tasks efficiently.

Exercise is very important! Exercise is the most important factor to facilitate food digestion.

Probiotics are the second most important factor the intestines need in order to keep the flow of food digestion unencumbered throughout the digestive system. Proper probiotic flora in the intestinal tract antagonize and assist in the cleansing of the unhealthy mucosal and fungal barriers that tend to obstruct the intestinal walls from proper food absorption.

---

[20]   Anthea Maton, Jean Hopkins, Charles William McLaughlin, Susan Johnson, Maryanna Quon Warner, David LaHart, and Jill D. Wright, *Human Biology and Health* (Englewood Cliffs, New Jersey: Prentice Hall, 1993).

The digestive tract is an awesome creation that God implemented in our body. It functions with hi-tech efficiency to absorb and distribute vitamins, enzymes, and minerals to their proper destination. If only one of the functions becomes defective, it creates acute health problems.[21]

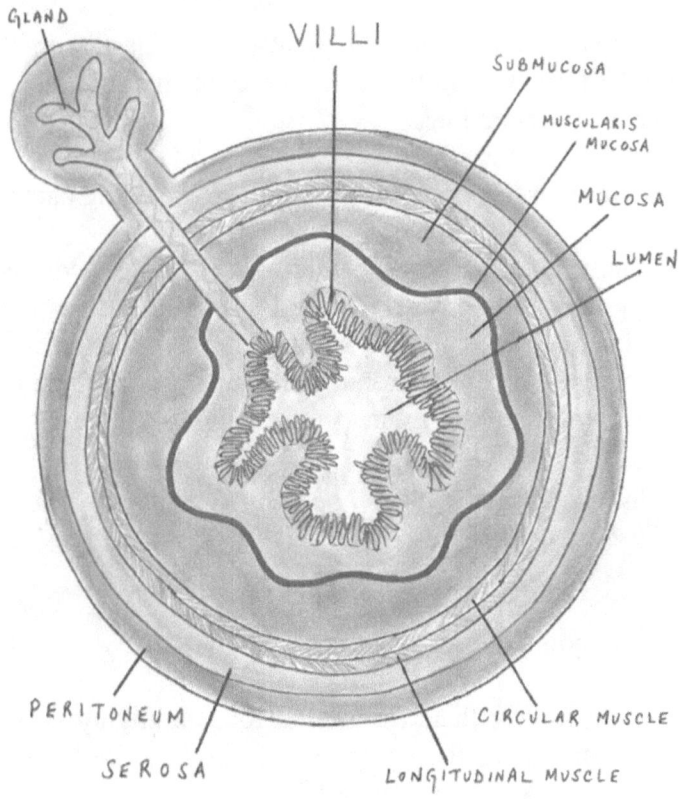

The Gut Wall (small intestinal wall - cutaway)

---

[21]   Orthodox Jews recite a blessing after defecating and urinating, praising God for His great wisdom in creating such a phenomenal harmonious ecosystem in our body.

Functions of the Gut Wall

The gut wall has amazing natural features that help the digestion and absorption of food into the intestinal tract. They are engineered in a fashion that ensures delivery of the food to their intended destination.

Peristalsis is the muscular movement in the digestive tract from the mouth all the way to the anus that forces the food downward via muscular contractions.

The circular muscles prevent the food from traveling backward.

Three muscles work together with coordinated contractions called "peristalsis" to propel the food through the digestive tract. The thickness of the muscles varies. They are thickened in the colon where the feces is hardened and needs more force to push the food down. They are thinner in the small intestine.

The mucosa lining contains the villi that trap and absorb minerals and vitamins into the bloodstream.

Serosa is the covering of the gut from the outer side to protect it from surrounding tissue.

We must be forever thankful to God for His mighty wisdom in which He structured the organs in our body to carry out their functions with ultimate precision.

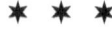

Probiotics Your Most Important Daily Supplement!

A prominent Naturopathic Doctor said: Daily probiotic supplements are more important than daily vitamins.

Let us understand the importance.

Healthy villi in your small intestine absorb and distribute the vitamins and minerals from the food you eat. If the food you eat does not supply ample amounts of nutrients needed to nourish your vital organs, you need additional supplements to accommodate your body's needs.

However, if your villi is clogged and glued from bacteria and fungus, the vitamins and minerals that you supplement are not absorbed and they bypass your small intestine as waste into your large intestine.

Probiotics battle the bacteria and fungus in your system an unclog your villi so that the nutrients can be absorbed to the liver, pancreas and vascular system and other vital organs.

The performance of your probiotics supersede all other supplements in order of priorities. All additional supplements are reliant on the healthy gut which is initiated through the functioning of your probiotics.

A Summary of the Functions of Probiotics

The healthy flora of probiotics accomplish three major functions:

A) Cleansing the digestive system
B) Supporting the immune system
C) Nutritional support of food digestion

A) They battle the fungus, parasites, and pathogenic bacteria that cling to the epithelial cells of your intestinal wall. They remove them and enable your digestive system to absorb the vital vitamins and minerals into your body's organs. In that phase, they act as cleansing agent.

B) They support your immune system, acting as a security force by destroying foreign pathogens entering the system. They supply energy to your digestive tract, which serves as the nerve center of your immune system. When your healthy flora diminish after antibiotic therapy, the good flora (probiotics) replenish the balance in your GI tract. With the help of good excipients, such as fruchtooligosaccharides (FOS) or prebiotics, the flora multiply and safeguard your intestinal tract and your entire immune system. They are equipped with memory sensors to search and destroy common invaders.

C) Food components that are difficult to digest and metabolize in the intestinal tract are supported by the intestinal flora. The flora help in breaking down the chemistry of the nutrients and aid in their absorption into the vital organs.

The Power of Probiotics

Defeating the Flu Now!

Believe it or not, probiotics are truly amazing!

Before I elaborate on the attributes of probiotics and how they work, I want to relate an amazing little story of the power that probiotics have.

John Taylor, ND, conducts nutritional courses across the United States together with leading authorities of nutrition and probiotics. He wrote a comprehensive book about probiotics and their functions, and it was called *The Wonder of Probiotics.*

He relates an amazing story about how probiotics saved the day for him when he had contracted flu symptoms.

His family ran an annual chili cookout competition among their friends in the neighborhood. The event was one day only and lasted for several hours. He woke up in the morning of that competition day with all the signs of the flu. He was nauseous and vomiting. He had diarrhea and was aching all over. It was approximately eight hours to the big event, and he was in a state of panic.

He was a probiotic specialist and believer. He immediately consumed 2.5 billion CFUs of a strong, potent probiotic containing five effective hard species and went to bed. Over the next eight hours, he continued taking a dose of 2.5 billion CFUs every two hours. By the time the first chili competitors rang his bell at 5:00 p.m., he was symptom-free. He had no more nausea, no more vomiting, no more diarrhea, and no more aching. He was a new person.

He did not want to press his luck too much, so he ate conservatively, only lightly sampling from the many different chilies. Throughout that night and the next day, he continued taking 2.5 billion CFUs every six to eight hours.

This story is just one example of the amazing effects probiotics can have on the health and fitness of your body in its entirety.

The same effects may apply to different ailments too.

CHAPTER THREE

Protecting the Immune System!
Your Amazing Immune System

Many different organs of your body have innate defenses against pathogens. These defense mechanisms, collectively, comprise your body's immune system.

Your skin is the first and foremost barrier repelling pathogenic organisms that seek entry into your body. The acidic pH levels of skin secretions inhibit certain pathogenic growth. Hair follicles of the skin secrete sebum, which contains certain acids that constrain the growth of fungus and pathogenic bacteria.

Your respiratory system, which thrives upon the oxygen you inhale, has its own defense mechanisms to thwart the entry of foreign pathogens. The sticky mucus in the respiratory tract repels many pathogenic organisms from entering your body. Other mechanisms, such as coughing and sneezing, assist in exhaling bacterial agents in the respiratory tract.

The Immune System Residing in Your Gut

The most amazing apparatus of your body's immune system is situated in your digestive tract (gut). Your digestive tract is equipped with a super-sophisticated system that discovers, identifies, and destroys pathogenic bacteria, fungus, and parasites that invade your intestines. The digestive tract also has an acute memory and tracking system that remembers and identifies the pathogens once they emerge again at later dates.

The healthy flora, or bacteria, in your intestinal tract are the food and fuel that nourish your body's immune system.

The healthy flora accomplish three extremely important functions that protect your body.

First, they defend against foreign toxic invaders, such as bacteria, fungus, germs, and viruses.

Second, they protect your body's ecosystem from pathogenic, degenerating, and malfunctioning cells.

Third, it gives nutritional support to your vital organs to aid in proper food digestion.

The mucosa, which lines the intestinal walls of the digestive system, secretes hydrochloric acid and protein-digesting enzymes that obliterate many pathogens.

Probiotic microorganisms assist the metabolism, digestion, and breakdown of minerals, vitamins, and enzymes into the body's organs. These healthy flora help the overall immune system of the body by identifying harmful toxins and pathogens, engulfing them, and destroying them. They assist your immune system through their ability to detoxify common allergens and carcinogens.

Anticarcinogenic Activity

Researchers have discovered that your body may produce up to ten thousand abnormal malfunctioning cells daily. Your immune system is trained to identify and destroy these malfunctioning cells before they can do any harm. When one of these abnormal cells is not destroyed immediately, it might break away and become carcinogenic. Once the healthy microorganisms defeat the invading toxins or pathogens, they have a memory that tracks and destroys them if they reappear again at any later time.[22]

Various disease-causing bacteria and fungus enter your digestive tract through the food you eat. The healthy microbiota or microflora serve as a security force to protect your intestinal tract and immune system from antagonistic pathogenic invaders and carcinogenic cells.

Researchers in the field of probiotic microflora and the human digestive system have been amazed about the awesome powers of the immune system that is situated in the digestive tract. Memorizing, identifying, and destroying antagonistic pathogens are inherent characteristic attributes of the gut that may rival the functions of the brain and the liver. The human brain has the ability to identify and memorize any potential maladies of the whole human body. The liver screens, filters, and destroys toxic and pathogenic elements that pose potential threats to the health and well-being of most organs of the body.

Even more exciting is the discovery of neuroscientist Candace Pert in her book, *Molecules of Emotion,* where she espouses the "feel good hormone" of the gastrointestinal tract. She claims that over 90 percent of the serotonin, which is the hormone that makes you feel good, is situated in the digestive system. Previous universal opinion held that serotonin is situated exclusively in the brain.

Hence the common saying, "I have a gut feeling."

I prefer to compare the abovementioned complex probiotic activity to that of a military operation. The probiotics formulas execute their duties like a probiotic militia. Their duties comprise two distinct military types of operations. I prefer to identify them as "Operation IAD," which stands for "identify, attack, and destroy." Their second duty I prefer to call "Operation AMVO," which stands for "absorb minerals and vitamins to vital organs." The metaphor

---

[22]   Jon Barron, *How Immunity Works* (Aug. 22, 2011).

that an army travels on its stomach may have more implications than is commonly understood.

Similar attributes to the aforementioned behavioral properties of probiotic flora were reported in the *New York Times* (Science Times) on September 13, 2011[23] as an amazing new breakthrough in the war on leukemia.

Researchers in the University of Pennsylvania outfitted T-cells to search, identify, destroy, and memorize cells of leukemia. The cells were equipped to recognize the carcinogenic cells, attack them, destroy them, and multiply, continuing to live inside the patient. The carcinogenic cells were wiped out. The T-cells were equipped to memorize them and destroy them again if they returned. Several patients of that successful experiment are now in remission.

Probiotics enriched with prebiotics perform similar functions: they multiply themselves and then they identify, attack, and defeat antagonistic bacteria and carcinogenic pathogens.

If and when the defeated cells reappear, even years later, your immune system will recognize them and destroy them with super speed. The second time they appear, the system acts even faster and stronger than before to destroy them.[24]

As I mentioned before, researchers have discovered that your body may produce up to ten thousand abnormal malfunctioning cells daily. If, and when, one of these abnormal malfunctioning cells breaks away and is not destroyed immediately, it might become carcinogenic. Your immune system is trained to identify and destroy these malfunctioning cells before they can do any harm.

We must be forever grateful to our Creator for implementing such an awesome immune system in our digestive tract that protects our health more than ten thousand times daily.

---

[23] "An Immune System Trained to Kill Cancer," *New York Times* (Science Times), Sep. 13, 2011, p. D1.

[24] Baseline of Health/Anatomy of the Immune System, Aug. 22, 2011.

Probiotics taken orally are compositions that have enhanced stability and potency under various storage conditions. The stability of these probiotic compositions is enhanced through the addition of various agents and excipients, such as prebiotics.

These probiotic formulas create a healthy environment in the GI tract, which strengthens the various systems of the body to perform at their maximum potential. The health and strength of your immune system is essential in the battle against pathogenic bacteria and carcinogenic cell aberrations.

Probiotics enriched with prebiotics replenish your immune system with the healthy flora needed in your digestive tract to protect your body 24/7.

CHAPTER FOUR

Probiotics for Fungal Infection Relief! Antibiotic Therapy and Infection Relief!

Yeast Fungus (Candida)

Yeast infections are extremely common, with over five hundred million cases reported yearly worldwide. Yeast infections are very annoying and cause a lot of discomfort, such as burning, itching, and twitching. The yeast fungus in the body weakens the outer skin, and it also can cause excessive staining.

Yeast infections, caused by the bacteria known as candida albicans (commonly called candida), colonize the urinary tract. Urinary tract infections (UTI) and yeast infections are caused by uropathogenic bacteria that enter the urinary tract.

Thrush in infants is similar to yeast infections in adults. Babies acquire thrush because their immune system is not strong enough to battle the candida growth inside their bodies. In elderly people, thrush may occur due to their weakened immune system on account of old age. Diaper rash is also a form of candida disorder. Probiotics taken by a nursing mother could alleviate the yeast and thrush infections. A bottle-fed baby can have probiotics emptied into his bottle to ward off the infection.

Candida is also the root cause of athlete's foot skin fungus, dandruff (or cradle cap in infants), some forms of eczema, and many other chronic epidermal sores or maladies. Fungal bacteria like candida thrive in dark and damp environments. Athlete's foot and yeast infections occur in similar dark and damp environments. The same holds true for dandruff of the scalp under your hair; the fungus thrives in a dark and moist environment.

Heightened acidic levels in the blood are the culprit that permits the fungus to grow. The fungus thrives and multiplies due to elevated acidic levels in the bloodstream. These acidic levels are measured biologically by a system called pH balance.

In 2005, a team of French researchers at the Institut de la Sante et de la Recherche Medicale found that pH levels were lowered when various strains of probiotics were consumed. The healthy (friendly) probiotic flora detect and destroy the fungus that creates yeast-related infections.

Probiotics with effective potent formulas of lactobacilli reduce or eliminate yeast infections. They have also proven to relieve or eliminate urinary tract infections (UTI).

A study conducted in 2002 by the Lawson Health Research Institute of Western Ontario, Canada, concluded that various lactobacilli strains of probiotics have the capability to help prevent infection by pathogenic bacteria in the urogenital and intestinal tracts.[25]

Controlling and Eliminating Recurring Ear and Yeast Infections

Children and adults who suffer from chronic ear sinus infections are normally treated with antibiotics, such as penicillin in the forms of amoxicillin or Keflex. The infection usually subsides

---

[25] Canadian Research & Development Center, Reid and Burton, 2002.

within a week to ten days, but it is not totally eliminated. Very often, the infection returns in a short period. The same is common with yeast infections.

The antibiotics battle the harmful bacteria effectively. However, at the same time they seriously damage the healthy bacteria or flora that help your body in the healing process. The immune system becomes weakened to the point where it is unable to sustain your healthy bacterial balance and the ear or yeast infection finds its way back into your body.

The National Primary Immunodeficiency Resource Center issued a letter of ten warning signs of primary immunodeficiency. Among the warning signs are four or more ear infections in one year; two or more months of antibiotics with little effect; and persistent fungal infection on skin.[26]

The same holds true with yeast infections. They keep on recurring after antibiotic treatment.

Probiotics are the answer. You must consume a considerable amount of probiotics after consuming antibiotics in order to regain the lost healthy flora from the digestive system. The probiotics replenish the energy needed in the immune system to stave off the pathogens that allow the infections to return. After antibiotic therapy, you should double your dosage of probiotics to counter the devastating effect of the antibiotics.

Nursing mothers consuming probiotics can positively affect and support their infants' immune system. Reports have shown that nursing infants were relieved of cradle cap, atopic eczema, and constipation when the mother or the child was fed effective probiotic formulas.[27]

---

[26]   Primary Immunodeficiency Resource Center, Jeffrey Modell Foundation, June 22, 2011 INFO4PI.ORG.

[27]   ProDermix Probiotic Research, "Effects on Nursing with Probiotics," Nov. 2010.

The probiotics together with the antibiotics effectively help to eliminate the yeast and ear infections. Consuming probiotics on a regular basis helps to control the bacteria from recurring.

Probiotics after Antibiotic Therapy

Ear infections and yeast infections recur commonly after a regimen of antibiotic therapy. As I mentioned earlier, the antibiotics destroy the harmful bacteria that brought on the infections. At the same time, healthy flora are also destroyed. The result is a weakened immune system, which leaves the inner organs vulnerable and susceptible to new infections. The same holds true for any probiotic regimen for any sickness. The immune system needs to rehabilitate the healthy flora that were depleted during the bout with the malady and the following antibiotic therapy.

It is very important to increase the amount of probiotics after the antibiotic therapy is over.

However, it is important to note that consuming heavy doses of probiotics while taking the antibiotics might be counterproductive. An adverse reaction could occur as the antibiotics fight the infection and at the same time, the probiotics battle the antibiotics, elbowing them out of the intestinal tract. That could effectively weaken the body's ability to eliminate the infection. It might actually prolong the time it takes to eliminate the infectious bacteria.

Healthcare practitioners and medical professionals suggest consuming probiotics during the antibiotics regimen. However, the probiotics must not be taken simultaneously with the antibiotics. It is advised to wait at least two hours between taking antibiotics and probiotics.

Increasing Probiotics after Antibiotics

A partial list of antibiotic drugs that require increased use of probiotics after their consumption

Dr. S. K. Dash, in his book *The Consumer's Guide to Probiotics,* lists more than thirty antibiotics that could need an increase in probiotics after taking those drugs. Some of those are below. (Only the generic names are listed.)

Amoxicillin
Ampicillin
Azithromycin
Ciprofloxacin
Clindamycin
Erythromycin
Levofloxacin
Neomycin
Ofloxacin
Penicillin
Quinolones
Sulfamethoxazole
Sulfasalazine
Tetracyclin
Tobramycin
Trimethoporim

CHAPTER FIVE

Skin Fungus Treatment!
Your Skin, the Body's Index of Health

As I mentioned previously, your skin is the primary organ of the body's immune system. Your skin is the first barrier against invading bacteria and fungus.

The skin is part of your body's integumentary system. The integumentary system is comprised of organs that protect your body's inner organs from damage. All major organs and cells of your body have outer layers that protect them from harm. The skin is your body's largest organ; it covers your entire body. It protects your innards from harmful toxins in the air and water. It serves as a security wall to restrain them from entering the body.

Your skin is a major gauge of your internal state of health. Many internal diseases manifest themselves by breaking out as rashes or eczema on the outer skin. Seldom are the rashes and inflammations of the outer skin caused by external diseases. The outer skin irregularities are indicators of internal toxification.

Your outer skin (epidermis) also serves as your body's toxic outlet by releasing pathogenic toxins from the body. When you contract an infection, your immune system fights the infectious bacteria and you begin to perspire. The perspiration exits through the pores of your skin, which is your body's method of cleansing itself and eliminating the infection.

Similarly, fungus inside your body travels to your epidermis, resulting in many types of candida fungus and eczema. Rashes and pimples on your outer skin are signs of toxicity inside your body. Athlete's foot fungus and yeast-related fungus (candida albicans) are among many different fungal diseases that strongly affect your outer skin.

When you cleanse your body from within through consuming the appropriate probiotics, most of your outer skin maladies will disappear. Of course, probiotics alone might not accomplish the task. You must follow a healthy diet of nourishment and keep a daily routine of exercise. Your skin will become healthy and most other internal maladies and disorders will improve. As a matter of fact, your entire gastrointestinal tract and most inner organs will become strengthened, and your overall health will show improvement.

Defeating Fungus of the Epidermis (Outer Skin)

Athlete's Foot Fungus, Cellulitis, Dandruff, and Jock Itch

Controlling or Eliminating Athlete's Foot

Athlete's foot fungus is classified medically as a dermatophyte. Tinea pedis is the fungus dermatophyte that causes athlete's foot. Tinea capitis causes ringworm of the scalp, and tinea cruris is the fungus related to jock itch.

These fungal dermatophytes attack dead cells of the skin and create a kind of dermatitis. Dermatophytes are also called ringworm.

Probiotic therapy, consuming probiotics on a regular basis, has been noted to ease and soothe athlete's foot.[28]

---

[28]   ProDermix Probiotic Research, attested to by Dr. Stanley Miller, DC.

Athlete's foot fungus is a very annoying skin fungus of the feet. When fungus is present in the digestive tract, the outer skin of the feet becomes tender. The skin itches and peels. Tinea pedis is the ringworm type of fungus that thrives in wet and damp places, such as locker rooms and swimming areas. The tinea pedis fungus enters the lacerated skin and causes athlete's foot to linger.

There are two basic types of athlete's foot fungus. One is called interdigital, which is between the toes of the feet. The toes become blistery and itch and burn. The skin begins to peel and the feet become very irritated.

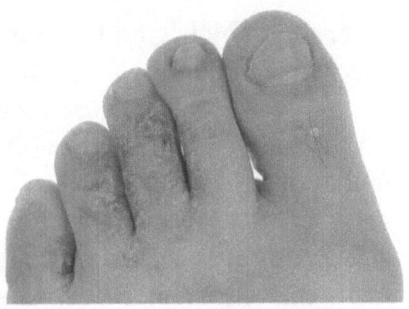

Interdigital athletes foot

The second one is the moccasin type, which manifests itself on the sole of the foot. The sole of the foot appears as a caked icing and the skin becomes hardy. Cracks appear on the bottom of the foot and walking becomes quite painful.

The athlete's foot skin disease has been noted to be held in check when potent probiotics are consumed as a health regimen on a continuous basis. The interdigital type of foot skin fungus, which is the lighter version of the fungus, shows relief much quicker than the moccasin type. However, over a longer period of consumption of probiotics, even the moccasin skin fungus softens and clears up. Skin calluses—hard, tough skin usually on the sole of the foot—also soften up sometimes, with continuous consumption of probiotics.

People have sampled potent probiotics to relieve their athlete's foot symptoms and were surprised by the outcome. Their feet became clear, smooth, and fungus free. As long as they continued consuming the probiotics, their athlete's foot fungus condition did not recur.[29]

The fungus of the skin apparently is related to the candida type of fungus (yeast related), and when it is rampant inside the GI tract, it tends to aggravate or weaken the outer skin. The tinea pedis fungus could not penetrate healthy skin that is not peeling or lacerated. Dermatophytes cannot invade or harm healthy skin. A healthy intestinal tract strengthens the outer skin.

It is interesting to note that athlete's foot fungus is mostly a male malady. Females seldom have the fungal problem. Women usually wear light and open shoes that don't enclose their feet entirely and they have more fresh air and ventilation. The athlete's foot scourge does not affect them that much.

Athlete's foot fungus got its name because athletes usually wear heavy shoes and socks that cause their feet to sweat excessively. The sweat and moisture of their feet cause the development of skin irregularities and soreness. The tinea pedis fungus enters the weakened, sore spots of the skin. Dandruff and yeast infections, which also occur in dark and moist environments, have similarities to athlete's foot.

It is important to note that there are hundreds of skin maladies and fungi. Some notable ones are psoriasis, eczema, and nail fungus. Some of them are very hardy and difficult to defeat. Athlete's foot has been identified as one that can be soothed with probiotics.

---

[29]   Prodermix Probiotics Research, November 2011.

Controlling or Eliminating Cellulitis

Cellulitis is a bacterial skin disease. The bacteria goes deep down into the skin. It may be contracted when athlete's foot fungus is uncontrolled. Cellulitis is a very painful disease. It can appear anyplace on the body. Most commonly, it appears on the lower parts of the legs. Light or deep red-colored skin tones are visible on the lower leg or foot. It is usually accompanied with very high fever with the body trembling and aching. The pain is excruciating.

Heavy doses of antibiotics are prescribed with constant bed rest. If it is not controlled, it can possibly lead to phlebitis (a blood clot, usually in the legs), which could be a life-threatening disease.

Probiotics taken regularly relieve the symptoms of athlete's foot and could help thwart the onset of cellulitis.

Controlling or Eliminating Dandruff

Dandruff is an annoying state of scaling of the scalp. Dandruff causes itching of the scalp and could eventually cause hair loss. It manifests itself as thin scales of skin that appear as white snow in your hair. Besides being a nuisance and quite uncomfortable, many times it is very embarrassing. It may also cause infection if your scalp bleeds from itching and irritation. Dandruff is a candida-related fungus of the outer skin.

The only known treatments for dandruff are shampoos that are fortified with chemical cleansing agents and vitamin formulas. These solutions are only temporary, since the dandruff comes back hours later.

Shampoos for cleansing or conditioning your hair could be very harmful. Health-care practitioners and many doctors are of the opinion that many of the ingredients contained in commercial shampoos are toxic and dangerous to your health. Some go so far as to claim that the toxic chemicals can severely compromise your immune system and adversely affect your reproductive health.

Several ingredients that are cited as toxic chemicals include the following:

- *propylene glycol* (also found in antifreeze), which may cause brain and liver damage
- *copolymer* (a petroleum derivative), which might be carcinogenic
- *imidazolidinyl urea,* which could cause nerve damage and skin irritations and is possibly carcinogenic

The list goes on and on. However, some are of the opinion that the amounts are only negligible and therefore are not harmful. The manufacturers of shampoo tend to tout the second opinion as being true.

Probiotic therapy holds promising solutions for dandruff sufferers who consume potent probiotics consistently. Dandruff of the scalp has declined or totally disappeared for many people consuming probiotics on a regular basis.[30]

Jock Itch

Jock itch is similar to athlete's foot since: it is caused by persistent sweating, and the fungus thrives in damp and moist environments. Men that suffer from athlete's foot commonly have jock itch.

An itchy red rash festers itself in the groin and surrounding area. It is very uncomfortable and sometimes quite embarrassing.

Fungal infections of the skin, such as jock itch, athlete's foot, and yeast infections, are caused by a weakened immune system and overgrowth of fungus in the intestinal tract.

---

[30]   Prodermix Probiotic Research, attested to by Dr. Stanley Miller, DC.

Eliminating body toxins with good probiotics assists the relief and gradual eradication of jock itch. It is not a quick fix and takes time for the probiotics to cleanse the intestinal fungus.

A healthy diet eliminating sugars and carbohydrates is a sure recipe for controlling candida-related fungus, which includes yeast infections, athlete's foot, and jock itch.

The probiotics function well with good diet and hygiene.

Acne Relief

A scientific study was conducted in UCLA University in Los Angeles regarding probiotics as a cure for acne.

Acne is a very common skin condition affecting forty to fifty million people in the United States. It manifests itself as unsightly pimples on the face. Some pimples are full of pus, those are referred to as cystic acne. Others that are simple puffy pimples are usually hormonal. And some are plain red blotches that may be called rosacea.

The study was published in February 28, 2013 in the Journal of Investigative Dermatology.

The researchers discovered that a certain bacteria caled 'P. acnes' is present in the skin of persons that are acne free. But persons suffering from acne lack that bacteria.

Their findings recommended using a probiotic cream which would address the P. acnes issue.

Topical cream may help the outer skin. However, treating the outer skin is only a superficial relief. The problem stems from within the body. Consuming probiotics orally could actually defeat the problem at its core within the body.

Although, no clinical studies were yet performed concerning the successful outcome of people consuming probiotics orally, results look promising. Many people suffering from acne were observed taking probiotics orally with gratifying results.

Atopic Eczema (Cradle Cap, Diaper Rash, Skin Rash, Etc.)

The College of Medicine at Swansea University in Wales (UK) studied the effects of probiotics consumed by pregnant mothers for reduction of atopic eczema and allergic sensitization in their children.

More than 450 mothers and their children were involved in the study that showed a 50 percent reduction of atopic eczema and allergic reactions in the first two years of their life.[31]

In other clinical studies, infants with atopic eczema, otherwise referred to as atopic dermatitis (a rash or pimples on the outer skin), have seen relief from their disorder with the supplementation of specific probiotic strains.[32]

Diaper rash is also a form of atopic eczema. It is also a candida disorder.

Cradle cap in infants is akin to dandruff in adults. It is a candida-related symptom.

General rashes of the skin in infants could possibly be soothed or relieved through probiotic consumption.

Probiotics consumed by a nursing mother or consumed by the infant in a bottle of juice or baby formula helps eliminate the candida conditions.

---

[31] Walesonline/news/50/20/2012/Probiotic Supplements for Pregnant Women.
[32] G. Ciprandi, A. Scordamaglia, et al., Effects of Treatment with Bacillus for Food Allergy, Chemioterapia, 1986.

CHAPTER SIX

Intestinal Tract Relief! Probiotics for Digestive System Enhancement

Probiotics Significantly Reduce Symptoms of IBS and Ulcerative Colitis

Inflammatory Bowel Disease (IBD) is a debilitating disease that is very common in the United States. Symptoms include inflammation of the large and small intestines, abdominal pain, diarrhea, and exhaustion. The two most common forms of IBD are ulcerative colitis and Crohn's disease. Over one million Americans suffer from this disease.

Irritable bowel syndrome (IBS) has similar symptoms to IBD. A patient suffering from IBS usually has the symptoms of bloating and cramping after eating a full meal. IBD can cause serious damage to the bowel. IBS irritates the nerves and muscles of the intestinal tract, but usually no harm is done to the bowels.

The National Institute of Health reported than one in five Americans suffers from the debilitating condition of IBS. It is a very common disorder diagnosed by doctors in the United States.[33]

Several studies were conducted in 2003 to assess the effects of probiotics on patients suffering from irritable bowel syndrome (IBS and ulcerative colitis). Dr. Stephen M Faber, a gastroenterologist from Elizabeth City, North Carolina, evaluated forty-four patients

---

[33]   Gary Huffnagle, PhD, *The Probiotics Revolution*, p. 117.

with IBS. Twenty were administered with probiotics only (10 billion CFUs twice daily). Twenty-four were given 500 mg of ciprofloxacin twice daily plus 10 billion CFUs of two strains of probiotics.

The Symptom Frequency Index (SFI), an indicator of pain and discomfort, decreased on average from 38 to 18.

The difference between the group given the probiotics with medication and the group that received probiotics only was negligible. The difference was recorded as statistically insignificant.

Ulcerative colitis also improved with probiotic therapy, according to a study done by Dr. Richard Fedorak, director of gastroenterology at the University of Alberta, Edmonton, Canada.[34]

Prodermix Probiotic Research tracked the results of several teenagers suffering from IBS who were taking probiotics to ease their pain and suffering. They consumed several capsules of 50 billion CFU probiotic dosage daily for several months and their pain subsided significantly. They were able to go off their medication. However, once they stopped, the probiotic regimen their symptoms reoccurred.[35]

Clostridium Difficile

C. difficile is identified as the bacterium that causes diarrhea and more serious intestinal conditions, such as Crohn's disease and IBS. It is a gram-positive, anaerobic, spore-forming bacillus that is responsible for the development of colitis.

---

[34] Medscape Medical News/Digestive Disease Week 2003, recorded by PPR, Nov. 27, 2011.
[35] Prodermix Probiotic Research, May 2012.

Lactobacillus plantarum and Lactobacillus paracasei, which are present in quality probiotic formulas, have been found to battle and destroy the C. difficile bacterium.

Helicobacter Pylori

H. pylori is the bacteria responsible for most ulcers and many cases of stomach inflammation (chronic gastritis). The bacteria can weaken the protective coating of the stomach.

The H. pylori bacteria invade the cell lining or mucus layer of the stomach. The bacteria weaken the stomach lining, and the natural stomach acids irritate the stomach wall until an ulcer develops. Peptic ulcers are believed to be caused primarily by the H. pylori bacteria.

It may also bring on colitis or other digestive maladies.

Lactobacillus casei, a strong strain that is used in many probiotic mixtures, has been found to antagonize and neutralize the H. pylori bacteria.

Constipation Relief

Constipation is not a disease. It is a digestive symptom that can lead to many diseases. The human colon handles the bulk of the waste of the food we digest. A healthy colon functions normally with two bowel movements daily.

Poor diet and lack of exercise cause the colon to become ineffective in eliminating the waste or fecal matter from your digestive system. The fecal matter then becomes hardened and clings to the intestinal walls. People who are constantly constipated may carry up to 40 pounds of toxic fecal matter in their colon. This heavy burden restrains the colon from properly eliminating the waste. It also obstructs the essential minerals and enzymes from penetrating into the proper organs.

The waste collected in the colon continuously toxifies the body and its organs. Excess fecal matter in the intestines can lead to diverticulitis, which is the formation of tiny sacs that store excess fecal mass in the colon wall. The fecal wastes stored in those sacs are difficult to clean out. As a result, they can become infected with fungus and bacteria. Fecal toxicity can bring on major health complications for patients with digestive disorders and for normally healthy people as well.

Fecal toxicity can weaken the heart. The brain can be adversely affected from the toxicity, causing foggy memory or senility. It can create stiffened joints and lead to arthritis.[36]

According to Dr. S. K. Dash, Ph D, research was done in the University of Turku in Finland, and it was found that certain probiotic strains helped to ease the frequency of bowel movements of many participants in the study.[37]

Probiotic formulas generally deposit healthy flora into the GI tract that actively destroy the bacteria that cling to the walls of the intestines. In that manner, they act as cleansing agents of the intestines. When they successfully clear the intestinal walls from the harmful bacteria, they also ease the elimination of waste through healthier bowel movements.

Diarrhea

Diarrhea in Greek means "flowing through." The WHO (World Health Organization) defines diarrhea as three or more watery stools in two consecutive days.

---

[36]   Colon Cleanse Information/toxic colon/12/12 2011.
[37]   S. K. Dash, PhD, *The Consumer's Guide to Probiotics,* Freedom Press, p. 55.

The American Society for Nutrition in 2007 reported on the effects of probiotics and prebiotics in treatment of diarrhea. The report was published in *Journal of Nutrition* in March 2007.[38]

The report concluded that probiotics have preventive and curative effects on several types of diarrhea. The same report also mentions the effectiveness of prebiotics to prevent strains of pathogenic bacteria, especially Clostridium (C. difficile) and diarrhea. The primary characteristics of prebiotics are their resistance to digestive enzymes in the human gut.

Dr. Stephen J. Allen, of the Swansea University School of Medicine, and his colleagues performed sixty-three studies with more than eight thousand participants regarding probiotics for diarrhea therapy. They found that probiotics with rehydration therapy was effective in reducing stool frequency in patients suffering from infectious diarrhea.[39]

In the University of California, at Berkeley, studies were conducted conclusively. It was found that certain probiotic strains can be helpful for treating acute diarrhea. A dose of 10 billion CFUs of Lactobacillus rhamnosus was used, among various other probiotics, with positive effects. In the case of antibiotic-treated diarrhea, such as C. difficile, they reported the significance of consuming at least 10 billion CFUs in a daily capsule to replenish the good flora (bacteria) that is destroyed by the antibiotic therapy.[40]

Controlling and Eliminating Colic Symptoms in Infants

An infant who is colic suffers extreme discomfort and agony. The child cries nonstop. The parents cannot get a good night's rest. The parents and the child remain tired and exhausted constantly, until the child finally outgrows the agonizing stage. It has a traumatic

---

[38] Jn.nutrition.org/content/137/3/803S.long.
[39] Medapagetoday.com/infectious disease/Nov/10/2010.
[40] Uhs.berkeley.edu/probiotics/09/29/09.

effect on the child and the parents. The household becomes very tense, and the parents' relationship suffers undue hardship.

Probiotics have been found to offer a solution.

A clinical study was performed by a group of researchers in Turin, Italy, regarding the relationship between colic and microflora. They discovered that colicky infants have a different pattern of microflora in their gut than noncolicky infants. Their intestinal tract is less frequently colonized with healthy Lactobacillus bacteria. Their GI tract possesses more nonprobiotic bacteria than usual. The study ascertained that a dose of probiotics laced with prebiotics can solve the problem.

The study was published in the *European Journal of Clinical Nutrition* in 2006 and involved close to two hundred babies with colic. The study found that the babies consuming the probiotic formulas laced with prebiotics were significantly relieved from their colic symptoms. More importantly, the other group of infants was treated with a regular formula of probiotics and simethicone drops, the standard colic treatment, but the first group strongly outperformed the latter.

A second study was conducted by the same group involving eighty-three infants who were having bouts of crying three hours or more daily, three to four times per week. After four weeks, the babies in the study that received the probiotic formulas reduced their overall crying to an average of fifty-one minutes per day, which is considered in the range of normal.[41]

Reducing Food Allergies and Asthma

A group of Italian researchers, in 1986, conducted a study concerning the effects of probiotics on food allergies. They concluded that certain strains of probiotics can reduce symptoms of some food allergies.

---

[41]   Gary Huffnagle, PhD, *The Probiotics Revolution* (Bantam Books, 2008).

In a study at the Seoul National University in South Korea, Bifidobacterium bifidum and Lactobacillus casei probiotic strains were administered to mice. The mice were divided into two groups, one being fed chicken egg whites and no probiotics administered. The second group received the same food with probiotics.

Their findings proved positively that the mice that were given the probiotic formulas had decreased allergic reactivity compared with the group that was not fed the probiotics.

Another study was done with infants taking Lactobacillus rhamnosus, and they also had lowered reaction to milk allergies.

These findings were published in 2005 in *FEMS Immunology and Medical Microbiology.*[42]

The College of Medicine at Swansea University in Wales (UK) studied the effects of probiotics consumed by pregnant mothers for reduction of atopic eczema and allergic sensitization in their children. The study found that babies assessed at two years of age who started taking probiotic supplements, had a reduced chance of allergic reaction to common allergens, such as cow's milk, eggs, pollen, and other dust-related allergies.

The same study addressed the symptoms of asthma related to atopic eczema. The study mentioned the probability of 80 percent of children developing asthma by age twelve if they had atopic eczema by age two. Obviously, if the probiotics can relieve atopic eczema, then asthma could be held in check. However, the study was not conclusive as to the real effects and benefits relating to asthma.[43]

---

[42]   Gary Huffnagle, PhD, *The Probiotics Revolution,* p. 412, 153.
[43]   Walesonline/uk/news/probiotic   supplements   for   pregnant women/05/20/2012.

Probiotics for Dieters and Dairy Consumption

Low-carb dieters are accustomed to eating lots of protein. Much of the protein comes from eating meat. Most beef today is treated with antibiotics and growth hormones. The end result of these treatments is the increase of parasitic bacteria in the intestinal tract. Probiotics are very important to counter the effects of the nonfriendly parasitic bacteria that enter your digestive system. You must feed your gastrointestinal tract with sufficient healthy bacteria for optimum health.[44]

Most diet programs cut out different types of foods that may have beneficial results for various organs. Supplements are very important to help replenish and/or replace the missing proteins, enzymes, or vitamins from the diet program. Although probiotics are not vitamins, they aid in their absorption into the body. Probiotics should be on top of the list of supplements necessary for the good implementation of any diet.

A recent study by health researchers claims that milk (and dairy products in general) consumption can be very damaging to your health. The antibiotics and growth hormones, including additional "vitamin therapy enhancements" for the cow's health (meaning the cow's increased production of milk for monetary gain not for the cow's health benefit), create toxins that endanger the endocrine glands in the human body.[45] Probiotics fight *these* toxins and pathogens and help to cleanse the gastrointestinal tract from the hormonal pathogenic and carcinogenic toxins.

Note: Yogurt bought in the store has some amounts of probiotics, but it does not supply a sufficient amount of probiotics needed to cleanse your digestive system or replace the healthy flora damaged by antibiotics.

---

[44]   Probiotics for Low Carb Dieters, Jon Barron Newsletter, January 2004.
[45]   Killer Milk, Healthier Talk (Newsletter), May 18, 2011.

Obesity Control (Weight Loss)

There have been studies suggesting probiotics as a means for weight control.

Now, there are nerves and hormones that send signals to the brain via the spinal cord when your gut has had enough nourishment and that signals your brain that you are satisfied. That means you may stop eating because you had enough.

The hormone peptide YY has been identified as a hormone produced in the digestive tract signaling that the meal is over and it inhibits appetite.

The nerves sending signals to the brain via the spinal cord are situated in the mucosal lining in the small intestine. However, when your epithelial wall of the small intestine is clogged up the nerve sensors and the corresponding hormones may not be able to relay the message, so you keep on eating. Once you unclog the villi through a routine probiotic regimen, the message may then get transmitted.

Thus, obesity may be controllable by following a prudent program of probiotic consumption.

Oral Hygiene and Bad Breath Improvement

The mouth is the aperture or the entrance to the digestive tract. The destructive bacteria in the digestive tract inhabit the gums and teeth as well. The billions of microbes from the digestive tract find their way up into the mouth, which is the orifice of the gastrointestinal tract.

Studies conducted in Turkey and Japan found that consumption of probiotics lowered the amount of cavities in the controlled group that took the probiotics. The same group also suffered less from bad breath.[46]

Health professionals suggest rinsing of the mouth and brushing teeth with a potent probiotic. The probiotic formula helps to neutralize the foul bacteria in the mouth.

Bad breath, otherwise known as halitosis, is attributed to either one of two symptoms. Bad breath may be caused because of decay in the gums or teeth. Another common cause of bad breath is from improper food digestion and/or reflux. In the latter symptom, gases from the improperly digested (or decaying) food produce a morbid smell that is emitted from the mouth. The odor is unpleasant and creates a very uncomfortable social experience for sufferers. Probiotics have had positive effects in eliminating bad breath.[47]

Probiotics help in the digestion of food in the GI tract and aid in the absorption of food particles and enzymes throughout the intestinal tract. They battle the pathogens in the GI tract that facilitate the foul smell and cause thrush and related gum diseases to plague the teeth and gums.

---

[46] Gary Huffnagle, PhD, *The Probiotics Revolution*, pp. 412, 195.
[47] Prodermix Probiotic Research, Jan. 15, 2012.

Increase the Power of Your Probiotics

Prebiotics can increase the potency of certain probiotic strains up to one thousand times, according to studies noted by researcher Jon Barron.

Some foods can decrease the power of the internal microbiota that thrive in your intestinal tract. Certain foods are prebiotic or create prebiotics that highly activate your internal army of healthy microbes.

Among those known to be sources of prebiotics are fruits, vegetables, and whole grains. Other known sources are red wine, tea, certain fats, herbs, spices, and dark chocolate. Your body cannot digest fiber, but probiotic microbes thrive and get rejuvenated with prebiotic consumption.

Prebiotics perform a dual mission. They feed the probiotica in your system and help them multiply. Some prebiotics slow down the antagonizing microbes that fight the good microflora.

CHAPTER SEVEN

Cholesterol and Glucose Control!

Reducing Cholesterol

Consuming probiotics on a regular basis in conjunction with necessary vitamins and minerals can bring tremendous benefits to a person's overall health.

Cholesterol is the buildup of fatty deposits on the walls of the arteries that can eventually block the flow of blood to the heart, and this can lead to heart attack. High LDL cholesterol is a serious sign of risk for heart failure.

Diet and exercise are very helpful to prevent the fatty deposit buildup. Probiotics may play a pivotal role in controlling cholesterol levels. Prebiotics have been researched and proven to lower LDL cholesterol.

Studies have been conducted to prove that certain strains of probiotics can lower the low-density lipoprotein (LDL) cholesterol.[48]

In *The Consumer's Guide to Probiotics,* a comprehensive book researching probiotics, is a study by Shinshu University in Japan that found that Lactobacillus acidophilus can improve the removal of cholesterol through stool excretion.[49]

---

[48] M. E. Sanders, Probiotics/Considerations for Human Health, 2003.
[49] S. K. Dash, PhD, *The Consumer's Guide to Probiotics* (Freedom Press), 78.

A study performed in the Jiangnan University in China tested 485 participants in thirteen clinical trials regarding the efficacy of probiotics to cardiovascular health. The study concluded that probiotics may have the ability to lower the LDL (bad) cholesterol and triglycerides significantly.[50]

Patients with high LDL cholesterol are usually treated with statin drugs. Statin drugs block the liver from producing certain enzymes that produce cholesterol. Although statin drugs are highly lauded in the medical profession for lowering levels of LDL cholesterol, some risks have been noted. Muscle pain in the arms and legs is a side effect of statin drugs in many patients.

Mevastatin is a commonly prescribed statin drug for lowering cholesterol (LDL) levels. Red yeast rice is a known source of statin. Mevastatin is found in red yeast rice. But taking red yeast rice as a natural substitute for medical drug statins does not eliminate the problem of muscle pain.

The Food and Drug Administration in early March 2012 directed pharmaceutical companies to add a few risks to the labels of statin drugs. Among the risks were memory loss, mental confusion, and diabetes alert.[51]

The clinical trials noted above show how probiotics can play a role in cholesterol count reduction. Probiotics do not interfere with any organ of the body. Their primary role is to strengthen the healthy microflora located in the digestive tract, and they cleanse the GI system from unwanted plaque. Naturally, fatty deposits that cause cholesterol to build up are held in check. No risks have been noted in the clinical trials.

When a doctor prescribes statin drugs for a particular patient, the doctor is aware of the information mentioned above. The doctor's opinion is of utmost importance. However, a person taking

---

[50]   Naturecity.com/Nutrition and Metabolic Cardiovascular Diseases, Sep. 17, 2011.

[51]   WEBMD/cholesterol mgmnt/2012/statin-risks-outweighed.

probiotics as a regimen for general health can probably see the cholesterol levels lowered and could ostensibly be weaned off some drugs.

Cholesterol and Triglycerides Reduced

A patient with cardiovascular issues, an avid consumer of probiotics and other supplements on a regular basis, visited his cardiologist for an annual checkup. The patient was not keeping a strict nonfat or low-cholesterol diet. Nor had the patient followed a stringent exercise program.

As a routine for the annual checkup, the cardiologist submitted blood samples to the lab.

The blood work showed good results. The LDL cholesterol was a bit elevated but in the normal range. The HDL cholesterol was at a very good level. The triglycerides and other vital statistics were at acceptable levels.

The cardiologist was surprised that, even without a proper diet and exercise program, the lab results were in the normal range. He was expecting vastly different numbers.

The catalyst was the consumption of probiotics and other beneficial supplements.[52]

It is really amazing how probiotic supplements can positively affect the overall health of the human body. Even more amazing is the fact that the supplements help the achievement of normal health without following healthy diet and exercise programs. (However, beware that no health professional espouses leading a lifestyle devoid of exercise and a good diet.)

---

[52] ProDermix Probiotic Research, December 2011.

Reducing Glucose Intolerance during and after Pregnancy

Women that have gestational diabetes mellitus (GDM) are seven times more at risk of developing type 2 diabetes than women that have a normal glycaemic pregnancy. GDM can convert into type 2 diabetes, which is associated with complications during pregnancy, premature morbidity, and mortality.

A study is presently under way in the Aga Khan University in Karachi, Pakistan, to determine the effects of Lactobacillus rhamnosus in regulating glucose metabolism in pregnant women.

Probiotics effects on glucose intolerance have shown positive results in pregnant mice. The immune regulatory properties in probiotics have been found to work effectively to control glucose metabolism. Lactobacillus rhamnosus is one the most effective strains of probiotics that have a proven record of safety for pregnant women.

In general, Lactobacillus rhamnosus is noted to be a most effective probiotic for many diseases and ailments.[53]

Reducing Blood Glucose Levels (Diabetes)

A study was conducted at the University of Otago, Dunedin, New Zealand, regarding the influence of probiotics on blood glucose levels in healthy and diabetic rats.

The study concluded that the diabetic rats fed probiotics saw their blood glucose level drop. However, the healthy rats did not see any differentiation in their blood glucose levels.[54]

---

[53] ClinicalTrials.gov/#NCT01436448, September 2011.
[54] PubMed/NCBI PMID:18777945 APR-JUN2008.

The study concluded that the administration of probiotics may be a beneficial therapy in the treatment of diabetes.

However, there have not yet been enough conclusive studies to ascertain the positive effects of probiotics on the glucose levels of human diabetics.

Reduced Risk of Kidney Stones

Kidney stones form as small crystals in the kidneys when certain acidic impurities enter the digestive system. Tiny kidney stones usually flush out of the kidneys during urination. Larger ones could be extremely painful and require liquids and strong medication to flush them out of the kidneys. Severe cases may require surgical procedures to have them removed.

Studies were performed in 2007 regarding the prevention of kidney stones. It was found that certain probiotics could effectively prevent the formation of kidney stones.[55]

---

[55]   Gary Huffnagle, PhD, *The Probiotics Revolution* (June 2007).

CHAPTER EIGHT

The Right Probiotic Formulas!

Why Are Some Probiotics More Potent and Effective Than Others?

Not all probiotics are created equal!

Some are more potent and effective than others.

There are three distinct qualities that qualify certain probiotics to be more potent and effective than others:

A) *Super strains*
B) *Prebiotic content*
C) *Genetic purity and quality control*

A) *Super strains*: Universally recognized super strains of hardy species of probiotic formulas play a pivotal role in the successful penetration of the flora into your digestive system. The supernatant (the media source on which the probiotic culture was fermented) is central to the ability of the formula to enhance the functioning of your immune system. The genus and strains of the probiotics are central to their effectiveness in supporting your immune system and the gastrointestinal functions. This information is usually mentioned on the product label or in the manufacturing company's brochure.

B) *Prebiotic content*: Probiotic formulas that contain fructooligosaccharides (FOS) or inulin are called *prebiotics*, which help promote the growth of healthy flora in the intestinal tract.

Studies have shown that certain strains of bacteria can increase their effectiveness up to one thousand times with the FOS known as prebiotics. Probiotics lacking this ingredient do not achieve the same potency.[56] The prebiotics are the tools the probiotics need to effectively accomplish their goal.

The Journal of Nutrition, published by the American Institute of Nutrition, reported a study of the effects of fructooligosaccharides (prebiotics) on the absorption of magnesium and calcium in the intestinal tract. The conclusion of that study showed that probiotics coupled with prebiotic ingredients cause a significant increase in the absorption of magnesium, potassium, calcium, and zinc into the intestinal tract.[57]

Probiotics laced with prebiotics are referred to as synbiotics.

Prebiotics can be classified as dietary fiber that is digestion-resistant. Prebiotics selectively stimulate the growth of only the beneficial bacteria in the gut and support the microfloral organisms, such as lactobacilli and bifidobacteria.[58]

Prebiotics are the food (nourishment) the probiotics need in order to multiply and survive in the intestinal tract. The prebiotics fortify the beneficial probiotic strains to perform at their utmost capacity. Prebiotics only nourish the healthy flora and do not supply any energy or power to the negative pathogens in the intestines.

Our poor eating habits and overall unhealthy diet cause food residue to adhere to the walls of the large intestine. The harmful bacteria cling to the intestinal wall and create blockages and polyps that obstruct the vitamins and minerals from being properly absorbed into the body. They also hinder the waste products from

---

[56] Jon Barron Report, The Probiotic Miracle, February 2011.

[57] E. Scharrer, T. Lutz, Effects of Absorption of Magnesium, etc., by the Colon, Z. Ernharungswiss, 1990.

[58] Modulation of the Human Gut Microflora, Tuhoy, Rouzaud, Bruck, Gibson, Curr Pharm Des, 2005.

being excreted through the bowels. These factors contribute to major problems and illness in the colon.

Prebiotics tend to destroy many of these harmful bacteria and help clean the intestines from these dangerous invaders. Probiotics that are outfitted with prebiotics in their formulas are very potent and effective in cleansing the GI tract and the colon from these pathogens.

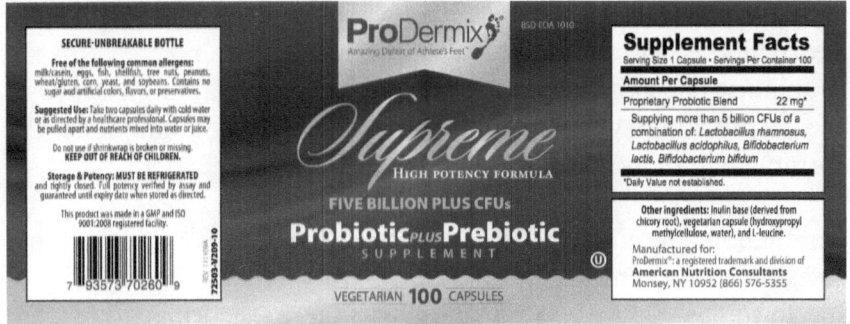

Probiotics with Prebiotics

Only the potent formula of probiotics with the exacting prebiotic compound has the capacity and potency to antagonize pathogenic colonies of bacteria. Prebiotics are the inert ingredients that help the host eliminate the adversarial hazardous bacteria that multiply in the gastrointestinal tract of the human body. As we mentioned before, the cells of healthy flora, in theory, engulf the pathogenic bacteria and deprive them of their pathogenic and carcinogenic capabilities.

Prebiotics are also reported to help with weight loss, keep LDL cholesterol levels low, keep blood sugars in balance, relieve constipation, and relieve symptoms of inflammatory bowel disease.[59]

---

[59] Natural digestion.com, December 2011.

C) *Genetic purity and quality control*: Certain exclusive manufacturing labs keep track of their inventory with a unique scientific-biological identification system. The various species and strains of probiotic formulas are categorized and classified with a genetic ID system similar to a human fingerprint. Each batch of probiotic flora is labeled scientifically with this genetic labeling to assure its purity and freshness.

This quality of certification assures the consumer that the quality of the probiotic formula was not compromised. The longevity of the shelf life of the formula, when stored according to the instructions, will definitely be prolonged. The potency of the probiotics depends on the quality and purity of the ingredients in the formulation. When manufactured under these conditions, the formula will deliver the intended benefit to you, the user.

Throughout the manufacturing process, the strains are tested and retested several times to ensure the viability, potency, and quality of the formulas. These labs operate under the most stringently sterile conditions, and their products are the most potent on the market.

Which Forms of Probiotics Are Best for You? Form and Formula

Probiotics that will effectively cleanse your digestive tract by eliminating pathogenic bacterial and fungal microorganisms should have the following qualities:

Form

First, probiotics are manufactured in four different forms: capsules, tablets, liquids, and powders.

Capsules are the most preferred form of supplementation. Capsules can usually be taken apart if one desires to halve the formula or divide the amount consumed. They also bypass the stomach bile and acids easier than liquid or powder (if the encapsulation is sturdy enough). Capsules are more apt to deliver the most benefits to your gastrointestinal system.

The liquid form of probiotic supplements is preferred for infants who cannot swallow capsules. However, it is much wiser and safer to empty the powder of the capsules into an infant's bottle of juice or bowl of cereal. The liquid form of probiotics cannot sustain their potency as long as capsules, and their shelf life is much shorter than encapsulated probiotics.

The tablet forms of supplements are ideal for children who don't drink bottles and the elderly who may have difficulty swallowing capsules.

The powder form is the least desirable. The powder can easily become contaminated once the bottle is opened and the contents become exposed to the open atmosphere. Once the powder is exposed to humidity, it may oxidize and compromise its potency.

Formula

The probiotics should include sufficient strains of Lactobacillus and Bifidobacterium species. The Lactobacillus species are active in the small intestine and the Bifidobacterium species perform their activity in the large intestine. Both species are important for a probiotic formula to greatly enhance the performance of the healthy flora in the gastrointestinal tract and beyond.

The following are important facts you need to know regarding the formulation of your probiotics:

1) The supernatant (media source of fermentation of the probiotic culture) is of nonallergenic nature and super strains. (This is usually noted in the manufacturer's brochure.)

FORMULA CONTENT

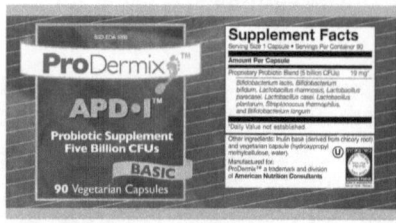
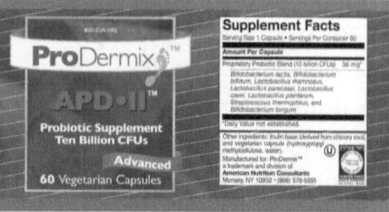
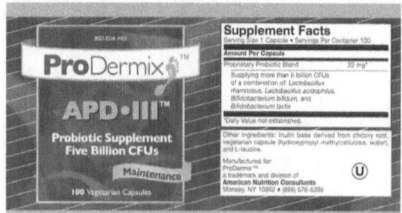
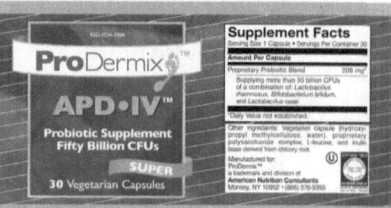

2) Live, healthy bacteria usually need refrigeration.

3) Quality probiotics contain prebiotics (inulin/FOS).

4) Effective potent probiotics are tested by independent labs to ensure that they are free of the most common allergens and of virus contamination.

5) Probiotics are routinely encapsulated to bypass stomach bile and acids.

6) Good probiotics are always independently tested for potency, purity, and virus contamination. (Potency and purity are the most significant factors in the strength and effectiveness of a probiotic formula. See copy of independent lab assay, page 83.)

7) The full stated potency of good probiotic formulas is guaranteed until the expiration date on the bottle. (Potent qualitative formulas tested by independent labs show billions of CFUs more than stated on the bottle. The range can be from three billion more to twelve billion more.)

8) Assays are submitted to independent labs for proof of expiration date potency.

9) Assays of expiration date potency are spot tested by agents of the Food and Drug Administration for veracity.

Which Probiotic Formulas Are Most Effective: One Single Strain or Multiple Strains?

Most probiotic formulas on the market today consist of multiple strains. However, most clinical trials and studies regarding the effects of probiotics are conducted with single strains.

The European Journal of Nutrition published a study regarding which types of probiotic formulas—single strains or multiple ones—are more effective. The study is entitled *Health Benefits of Probiotics: Are Mixtures More Effective Than Single Strains?*

The study concluded that mixtures of various strains of probiotics had a definite synergistic effect in the inhibition of the growth of pathogens and atopic dermatitis. Of sixteen studies, twelve showed the mixture of strains to be more effective than one single strain.

The studies were quite complex and in-depth pertaining to many different ailments and pathogenic bacteria. The studies encompassed the following: IBS syndrome, colitis, pouchitis, H. pylori treatment, atopic dermatitis, acute diarrhea in children, respiratory tract infections, and much more.

The same studies also pointed to the synbiotic effect of probiotics and prebiotics as being an effective tool to increase the probiotic potency and presence while defeating pathogens in the intestinal tract.[60]

Independent labs analyze the content of probiotics according to their microbiological form and content. It is interesting to note that when a multistrain probiotic formula states the CFU count on the bottle, the aggregate count of all the strains is mentioned. The individual strains are not dissected and enumerated. The reason for that is because biologically, under the high-powered microscope,

---

[60]   *European Journal of Nutrition,* 2011, 50:1-17 & PubMed database.

it is difficult even for the most professional lab technician to ascertain the difference between the strains.[61]

How Often Should You Consume Probiotics?

Every person has approximately four hundred different species of healthy beneficial microorganisms that flourish in the intestinal tract.[62] These species aid in the digestion and absorption of the vital vitamins and minerals into your organs. The majority of these species are not indigenous to the GI tract. They are not natives or inhabitants of the digestive tract and do not remain there indefinitely.

Many factors contribute to the decline and compromise of these friendly beneficial flora.

1) Age—As you age, the colonies of healthy bacteria also age and their vitality diminishes.
2) Antibiotics—Consumption of antibiotics destroys intestinal flora.
3) Chemicals—Chemicals in drinking water and septic seepage into the underground sources of water and vegetation bring bacterial fungus into your daily food consumption. The healthy flora get compromised.
4) Diet—The standard highly processed foods of the Western diet highly restrict the healthy and plentiful colonization of these important healthy flora.
5) Hormones—Additives to meat and dairy products compromise healthy flora.

Vegetarians and people consuming plant-based diets have a high rate of colonized lactobacilli, such as L. plantarum, L. rhamnosus, and L. acidophilus.

---

[61]	GBL Labs, L. Moyes, Ogden, Utah, May 2012.
[62]	Over one trillion units of microbiota inhabit the intestinal tract. The number of species is over four hundred.

People residing in Western countries do not retain enough healthy flora to sustain their probiotic balance. Probiotics must be replenished on a daily basis in order to be effective. Therefore, probiotics must be consumed daily.

The benefits begin to take effect immediately.

Realizing actual improvement to your digestion, heartburn (acid reflux), regulated bowel movements, yeast overgrowth, and epidermal disorders may take some time. However, within two or three weeks after taking an effective probiotic formula, you should see improvement.

To heal the gut (intestines), it may be necessary to persistently consume ample amounts of probiotics for many months. However, a super-healthy gut takes lots of time and effort to realize. A proper diet and daily exercise are very important, when they are combined with a strict regimen of probiotic formulas.

The advantages and benefits of probiotics are vast and tremendous. They support the health of most organs of your body. Plus they antagonize many pathogens and battle unhealthy bacteria within and outside the human body. The immune system and the liver are supported through the intake of the healthy flora. Yeast infections (candida) and urinary tract infections (UTI) are soothed and eliminated through the consumption of probiotics. Foot skin fungus (athlete's foot) and several other noted skin disorders have been known to disappear when probiotics are taken regularly. The list goes on and on.

The longer you consume probiotics, the more beneficial it is to your overall health and well-being and good quality of life in general. Even without any negative symptoms of any allergies or skin fungus, probiotics tend to cleanse your inner systems of the body for healthy consumption of food and normal absorption of vitamins and minerals into your body's organs.

Suggested Daily Dosage

Your health-care professional is most qualified to recommend which dosage is best for you. A conclusive study has not yet been done to establish the necessary dosage for various symptoms. Every person is different and must be evaluated on an individual basis.

As a rule of thumb, once your body is attuned to consuming probiotics, two capsules of a potent formula containing 5 or 10 billion CFUs should suffice for maintaining a healthy gut.

Some individuals have a very delicate stomach and could get diarrhea or upset stomach when beginning a strong probiotic. If and when you have these symptoms, you should stop taking the probiotic for several days and then begin again with a half capsule of the 5 billion CFUs. The smaller dosage should get your system habituated to the formula, and after normal stomach behavior, you could up the dosage to 5 billion or more gradually. The fact that the digestive tract reacted adversely to the formula proves that the probiotics are performing and functioning.

You should always seek the advice of your health-care professional in such instances. A large dose of strong, potent probiotics could cause discomfort to some people.

Sufferers of acute conditions of IBS, colitis, dermatologic eczema, or psoriasis could consider a highly potent formula containing 50 billion CFUs. The daily dosage could be from one to five capsules. Consult with your health-care professional before consuming such a high dosage.

Digestive System Cleanse and Detoxification

Probiotic formulas consisting of 50 billion or more are suggested for digestive system cleanse and/or detoxification once every six months. These capsules may be taken together with your regular probiotic therapy regimen of 10 or 20 billion CFUs.

Detoxifying your digestive system twice yearly is a good practice to keep many maladies and disorders from plaguing your body's health. (See Chapter Five, titled "Skin Fungus Treatment! Your Skin, the Body's Index of Health," p.41.)

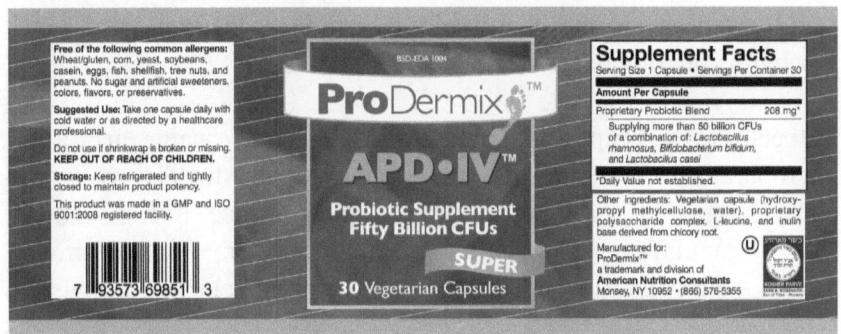

Sample of 50 Billion CFU label

How Are Probiotics Manufactured?

Probiotics can be produced naturally, the old homemade way, or biologically in a controlled laboratory environment.

Natural probiotics are created through fermentation of certain foods. Beets and cabbage are commonly used in many countries and cultures around the world to produce healthy food that contains healthy bacteria or flora.

Beets are cut up and soaked in barrels of water at room temperature. The barrels are covered with towels to keep them warm several weeks until they produce a rich lather of fermentation. The lather is healthy flora that destroys salmonella, clostridium, and many other pathogens and fungus.

A similar process is done with cabbage until it becomes sour. It is called *sauerkraut*, which in German means "sour cabbage."

Laboratory-manufactured probiotics are processed by isolating certain bacteria yeasts and molds from various plants, fruits, and vegetables.

In the 1980s, two well-known microbiologists, Gorbach and Goldin, discovered Lactobacillus rhamnosus. They obtained their original cell specimen samples from the flora of the digestive tract of a human being.[63] The strain was labeled Lactobacillus rhamnosus, GG, in honor of the two biologists. Other labs followed with production of similar specimen samplings.

Lactobacillus rhamnosus was identified as a very hardy species with qualities to defeat many pathogens. It has taken a front position in the formulas of probiotics, ahead of Lactobacillus

---

[63] Hence the term *human probiotics.*

acidophilus. Its performance is similar to Lactobacillus acidophilus plus much more.

Some refer to these specimens as human strains. However, it is generally accepted in the probiotics industry that all probiotics, whether from human or plant origin, are considered human strains since they are compatible and beneficial to humans.

The original flora are usually stored at freezing temperatures: −70 degrees Fahrenheit. The additional flora are produced in vitro. A minute amount, as tiny as a milliliter of the microbes of the above media, is placed upon a petri dish with fermentation media until a considerate amount of bacteria grows alongside it. It is then put into centrifuges to accelerate the fermentation process.

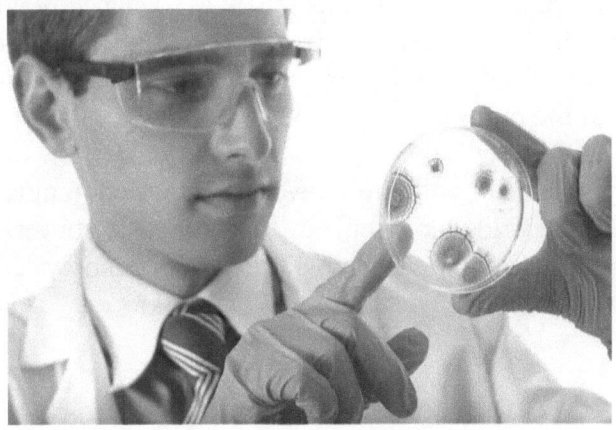

Microbiologist studying Petri-dish

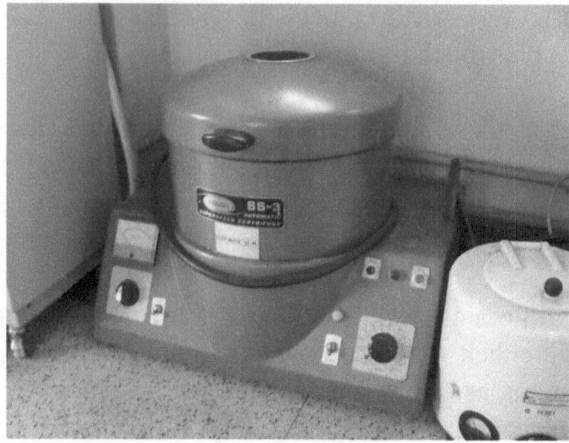

Small centrifuge

Once the bacteria have fermented and produced volumes of additional bacteria, they are freeze-dried and stored in large bins. Certified microbiological chemists count and control the potency of the probiotics.

Some of their nutrients are converted into lactic acids. Lacto-bacillus and Bifidobacterium are bacteria that convert certain nutrients into healthy lactic acid. They are commonly referred to as LAB or lactic acid bacteria.

CHAPTER NINE

Safety of Probiotics!

How Safe Are Probiotics?

Are Probiotics Approved by the FDA?

Probiotics are not subject to FDA approval since they are natural supplements and they are not drugs. However, they are considered "GRAS" (Generally Recognized As Safe) by the FDA. This classification is given to natural products that have been used safely for many years. However, the Food and Drug Administration does check the veracity of claims made by supplement-manufacturing laboratories.

Are Probiotics Safe for Infants?

Are Probiotics Safe for Pregnant Women?

Are Probiotics Safe for Nursing Mothers?

Are They Safe for Patients on Medication?

The answer to all of the above is *yes*!

Probiotics are similar to what all healthy people have in their in the digestive system: healthy flora (bacteria). As I discussed in the previous chapters, many factors cause the healthy flora to diminish and disappear from the intestinal tract. In order to maintain your healthy digestive system, you must replenish the good bacteria on a daily basis.

Infants are born with a weak immune system. The breastfed milk from nursing mothers is full of super-healthy flora and other vitamins that nourish the infant and support the immune system. It is very helpful for nursing mothers to consume probiotics in order to nurture the overall health and well-being of her child and herself.

The same holds true for pregnant women. The probiotics support the digestive tract of the mother and assist in the nourishment of the fetus in the womb.

Yeast infections are quite prevalent in pregnant women. Probiotic intake has relieved the occurrence of candida during pregnancy for many women.[64]

Nursing mothers have seen their infants' eczema disappear after consuming certain probiotic formulas. The disappearance of infants' cradle cap was also reported after consuming probiotic formulas.[65]

In summation, probiotics are safe and recommended for people of all ages in most conditions.

Could Probiotics Be Unsafe?

Clinical studies have shown that besides being very beneficial to your health, probiotics are exceptionally safe.

In 1999, hundreds of clinical trials of probiotics effects were performed on subjects ranging from preterm infants to elderly adults. The trial subjects ranged from healthy individuals to

---

[64]   Prodermix Probiotic Research, May 2012.
[65]   Prodermix Probiotic Research, Nov. 2010.

chronically ill patients. There was not a single adverse event reported.[66]

In 2010, the American Journal of Clinical Nutrition reported on clinical trials where probiotics were administered to health-compromised persons receiving nutritional support. There was no instance of increased infection.[67]

In addition to the above studies, probiotics have been shown to be helpful and effective in patients undergoing radiation therapy and chemotherapy.

A report of possible infection that may be caused by probiotics was reported by the *Natural Health Remedies* newsletter by Jon Barron. The report dealt with one specific strain only: Lactobacillus acidophilus. Lactobacillus acidophilus is a highly celebrated strain of probiotics and the first known and foremost probiotic.

People that have had injuries or illnesses affecting their intestinal wall are at risk. It can also cause infection of the heart lining in adults. Also patients taking prescription drugs, such as prednisone, could be vulnerable to infections. (see page 96)[68]

However, there are many effective probiotic formulas available today that have superseded acidophilus that are very potent and effective without the known side effects or harmful properties, and their ingredients do not contain acidophilus.

---

[66] Probiotic spectra of lactic acid bacteria/*Critical Review Food Science Nutrition* 1999;39:13-126
[67] *American Journal of Clinical Nutrition* 2010;91:687-703/Safety of probiotics in patients receiving nutritional support.
[68] Jon Barron's newsletter, July 2012.

Independent Lab Testing of Stated Potency and Potency at Expiration Date, and Freedom from Allergens

Expiration Date

The Food and Drug Administration provides guidelines to the nutraceutical industry known as "GMP" (good manufacturing practices).

The Food and Drug Administration recently implemented a new, stringent regulation regarding the stated expiration date of supplements. Supplements that state an expiration date on the bottle must submit assay tests to third-party labs to ascertain the veracity of their potency until the expiry date. The FDA conducts spot inspections at GMP labs to check their accuracy.

A strong, reputable, potent probiotic usually displays an expiration date.

Reputable labs *guarantee full potency until expiration date.*

Potency and Freedom from Allergens

The potency of probiotics manufactured by reputable laboratories is normally verified by third-party independent labs. The testing procedure is an accepted industry standard. The strains are usually tested for three basic criteria:

1) Potency strength
2) Free of virus contamination
3) Free from common allergens

The independent laboratories issue certificates of assay and analysis. The certificates ascertain the veracity of the amount of potency printed on the label and the absence of many viruses, allergens, and bacteria.

Among others, the labs test for any presence of:

E. coli
Mold
Yeast
Staphylococcus aureus
Pseudomonas aeruginosa
Salmonella spp.
Enterobacteriaceae
Milk allergens

A reputable manufacturer of probiotics should be able to provide proof of independent assay and analysis of its products.

INDEPENDENT LAB ASSAY

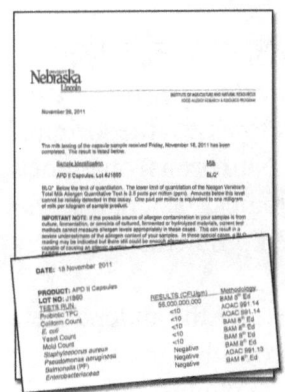
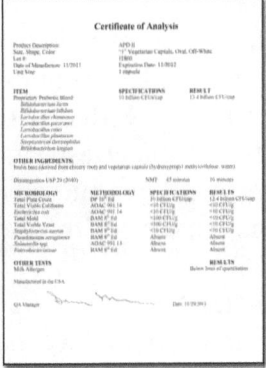
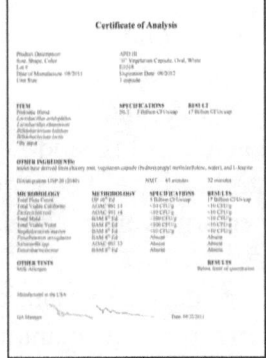

Patented or Certified Strains

Are patented or certified strains of probiotics superior to others on the market?

Several probiotic manufacturers market their probiotics as certified strains with code numbers, such as Lactobacillus GG, DDS1, or LP52.

Lactobacillus GG is a patent held by Culturelle Corp. Gorbach and Goldin are the microbiologists that discovered Lactobacillus rhamnosus, which the Culturelle company coined LGG in honor of its microbiologists. Other reputable manufacturers use different labeling and numbering for their own control and identification.

The nomenclature and numbering of strains are means of identification for marketing purposes only. The identification serves the purpose of showing exclusivity in the marketplace rather than to prove quality and potency.

Lactobacillus acidophilus is the first and foremost known probiotic that was acknowledged and used more than fifty years. It is the probiotic identified by Dr. Metchnikoff in 1908. Microbiology has advanced since then to produce many new strains that perform well in alleviating a plethora of health symptoms.

Lactobacillus rhamnosus is one of many probiotics manufactured by probiotic manufacturers and laboratories worldwide. It is a truly effective and potent probiotic. Perhaps it surpasses the original Lactobacillus acidophilus in many aspects. Numerous other new strains have been developed by microbiological scientists that perform well in alleviating many health-related problems.

The most important criteria for potent strains are the independent lab reports the manufacturer can produce to prove that the strains of probiotics it produces are of high quality and guaranteed potency.

Samples of supporting lab reports and independent lab assay certificates are illustrated above.

Measuring Probiotic Potency

What Is the Connotation of Colony-Forming Units (CFUs)?

The strength and potency of probiotics are measured in units known as CFUs. Microflora are the healthy, active bacteria residing in your intestinal tract that proliferate into colonies of multiple units. These colonies are called colony-forming units.

The measurements are usually noted in high visibility on the bottle, which denotes the amount of miniscule microbial units of microflora that mutate into multiple units in the intestinal tract. These microbial units measure in the millions and billions. Their numbers are counted and calculated only under super-microscopically controlled conditions utilized by biological technicians who study, understand, and are qualified to configure microbiological calculations.

A healthy colon has anywhere from one hundred billion to one trillion (one thousand billion) microbial units of healthy bacteria (microflora) per milliliter (approximately one-fifth teaspoonful). Their presence can only be detected through ultra-powerful biological microscopic identification. The measurements of the billions of units are categorized as CFUs.

It is interesting to note that when a multistrain probiotic formula states the CFU count on the bottle, the aggregate count of all the strains is mentioned. The individual strains are not dissected and enumerated. The reason for that is because biologically, under the high-powered microscope, it is difficult even for the most professional lab technician to ascertain the difference between the strains.[69]

---

[69]   GBL Labs, L. Moyes, Ogden, Utah, May 2012.

There are specialty labs that conduct DNA-type testing to assure that a named strain is actually the correct one.

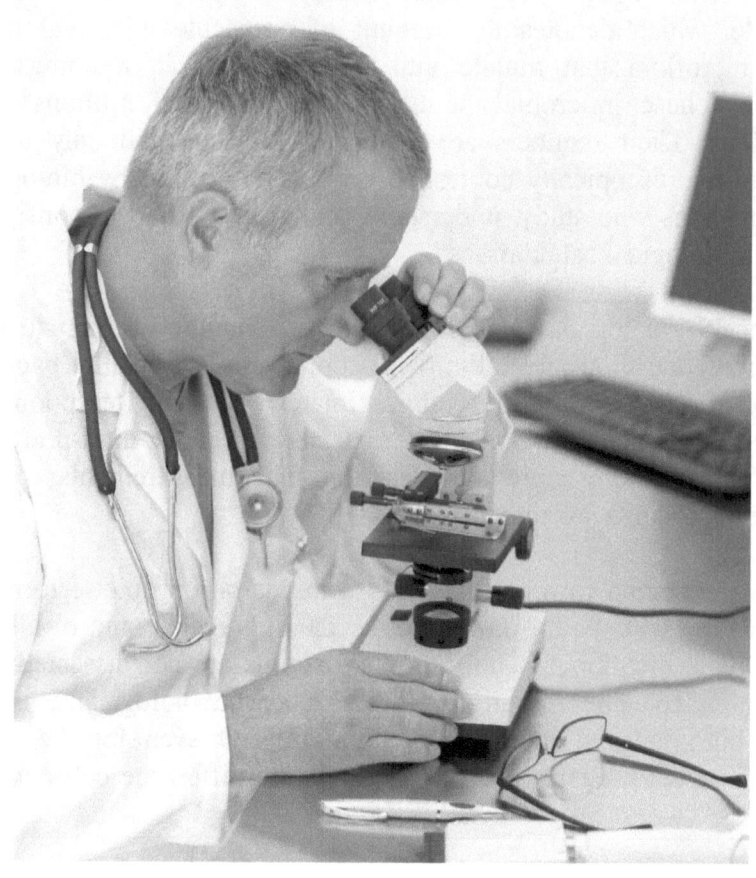

Microbiologist studying probiotic potency count (colony forming units-CFU's)

CHAPTER TEN

Live Probiotics

The Live Probiotic Army

Cool Temperature Keeps Them Alive

Remember the old adage "an army runs on its stomach"? Well, if your stomach and intestines are healthy, then you have an army of trillions in your digestive tract that offer you protection.

The "probiotic army" boosts your energy, your immune system, and helps digest your food and distribute the vitamins, minerals, and enzymes to your vital organs.

This "army" is only powerful and successful when its microflora are live. Live microflora means natural, fresh probiotic flora without any artificial additives.

The only practical and correct method of keeping probiotics live is through refrigeration. (Hardy, potent probiotic formulas can usually withstand temperatures up to 68 degrees Fahrenheit up to a maximum period of two weeks without refrigeration. This information is important for travelers.)

Innovations, such as chemical compounds and additives or preservatives, act as artificial sustainers of life. It is similar to keeping a patient alive with life support, such as respirators or heart-pumping equipment. The patient is kept alive but has no power or energy to fight or battle any aggressors.

Live probiotics are the fighting troops that battle and antagonize the harmful bacteria and pathogens that enter the digestive tract. If their liveliness is compromised through artificial means, they become handicapped in their battle with the antagonizing bacteria.

Probiotics fight and struggle relentlessly in your intestinal tract to protect the good flora and destroy the harmful pathogens and bacteria.

Prebiotics are added to probiotics to cause the probiotics to proliferate and multiply. Several species are known to multiply up to one thousand times.[70] Live microflora are nurtured by feeding on the prebiotics.

Live probiotics (or microflora) support your overall health and strengthen your immune system, by identifying and destroying harmful toxins and pathogens entering the gastrointestinal tract. They cleanse the intestinal wall and remove the fungal and parasitic cells that cling to them. They strengthen your intestinal microflora and relieve constipation, diarrhea, and other digestive irregularities.

The probiotic battle can only be won with live and effective microflora.

Stability of Probiotics

Shelf Life

A major disadvantage of many probiotic formulations on the market is their poor shelf life.

As I mentioned before, refrigeration is vital in the scientific art of prolonged shelf life of probiotics.

---

[70]   Jon Barron Report, The Probiotic Miracle, February 2011.

The live colonies of bacteria of Lactobacillus and Bifidobacterium can only survive in a cool, temperate environment. Many celebrated brands of probiotics claim "potency guaranteed at time of manufacture." Independent lab tests tracked some of them several weeks later and found that they had lost up to 95 percent of their original potency.[71]

Unrefrigerated probiotics cannot sustain *live* bacteria. Probiotic flora must be kept at a temperature of 35 to 49 degrees Fahrenheit in order to remain live and viable. Marketing people love the convenience of probiotics that don't need refrigeration, because it is easier to promote. However, the most potent formulas are those that are truly *live* in their natural state with no added artificial, man-made preservatives.

Refrigeration is of utmost importance to maintain the full stated potency of the probiotics. However, tests were conducted to check their potent stability at room temperature (50 to 68 degrees Fahrenheit). Probiotics of high purity with species of confirmed quality content were found to have maintained their potency without refrigeration up to several weeks. Their potency held up well. There was a maximum loss below 5 percent.

Additionally, sophisticated labs add sufficient overage of formula content to ensure against potential loss of the stated potency on the bottle. While this process ensures stability up to the expiration date, it also reinforces its stability in case of nonrefrigeration for a short period. However, over a longer period of time in an unrefrigerated state, the loss of potency would accelerate.

Probiotics in Glass or Plastic Bottles?

The live, healthy bacteria which comprise probiotics usually live in the absence of oxygen (anaerobic organisms). Being exposed to air is not good or desirable for their viability. Moisture is even worse

---

[71]   Barron Report, The Probiotic Miracle.

for their existence. Packaging is of utmost importance to assure the absence of air and moisture.

Glass bottles seem to be less apt to let in air or moisture.

However, tests have proven that high-density plastic (high-density polyethylene) bottles that are used for vitamins and probiotics have the same effect. The difference is negligible. Every bottle contains a desiccant or two to absorb the moisture.

A secure, unbreakable bottle has its own advantages.

CHAPTER ELEVEN

Benefits of Probiotics!

Longevity of Life and a Healthy Gut Strengthening Your Immune System

The great sage and physician, Maimonides, states in his master works relating to personal health and well-being that the fundamental causes of most sicknesses are attributable to bad eating habits and indigestion.[72] In other words, a healthy gut is a healthy human being.

However, it is important to note that in the same paragraph, he also states, "Even if one eats the finest foods but leads a sedentary lifestyle and does not exercise, that person will become sick and frail." There is no doubt that the probiotic "magic" cannot deliver its benefits to your digestive system if you consume all the wrong foods and don't exercise. Probiotics are only supplements to nutrition, but they are not, and are not intended to be, magic pills.

Healthy flora in the digestive tract protects the intestines from invading pathogenic bacteria. Thus, they strengthen the immune system.

When the intestinal tract is well balanced with the necessary probiotics, the immune system can successfully stave off the following known pathogenic bacteria and fungus. Such a well-balanced immune system:

- Protects against food poisoning

---

[72]   Maimonides/Mada/Daos/Chap. IV/para/15.

- Protects against stomach ulcers
- Immunizes against lactose and casein intolerance
- Inhibits digestive cancers
- Diminishes and eliminates yeast infections (i.e., candida and vaginosis)
- Improves absorption and generation of B vitamins internally
- Boosts energy
- Supports immune system
- Increases overall health

Consuming potent probiotics regularly contributes to a healthy intestinal tract (gut). Longevity of life and good health depend heavily on the superb functioning of the digestive system.

Boosting Your Energy

A healthy gut makes a healthy human being. It also makes a strong and energetic human being. Consuming probiotics on a constant basis increases and strengthens your energy.[73] One of the positive side effects of taking probiotics for soothing of UTI or yeast infections is the increased energy feeling. A second positive side effect is the impressive boost in the "feel good hormone." [74]

---

[73]   Prodermix Probiotic Research, May 2012.
[74]   See Chapter Three: "Anticarcinogenic Activity."

Benefits Attributed to Probiotics (Symptoms Relieved)

Fifty-Nine Known Benefits! There Are Many More!

Probiotics marketed today are extremely beneficial to the gastrointestinal tract, the immune system, and most organs of the human body.

The benefits of various species of modern-day probiotics (varying among different species and their respective potency and formulation) form a quite long list.

Fifty-Nine Benefits Attributed to Potent Strains of Pure Probiotics

Absorption of vitamins and minerals (See page 11, 25)
Acid reflux (See page 73)
Allergies (food allergies) (See page 54)
Anticarcinogenic activity (See page 32)
Antibiotic therapy (strengthen immune system) (See page 39)
Athlete's foot (See page 42)
Bad breath (See page 57)
C. difficile (bacteria causing colitis and IBS) (See page 50, 53)
Candida (albicans) (See page 36)
Cellulitis (See page 45)
Colic baby (See page 53)
Colitis (See page 49)
Constipation relief (See page 51)
Cholesterol (See page 60)
Cradle cap (See page 48, 80)
Crohn's disease (See page 49)
Carcinogenic activity defense (See page 32)
Cervical skin erosions (excessive staining) (See page 36)
Dandruff (See page 45)
Detoxify digestive tract (See page 74)
Diabetes support (See page 63)

CHAPTER TWELVE

Probiotic Strains and Formulas!

Popular Potent Probiotic Strains of Bacteria

Lactic acid bacteria (LAB), known as the Lactobacillus varieties of probiotic species, are predominantly found in the small intestine. Among the most popular potent species and strains of LAB probiotics that are included in various supplements are Lactobacillus acidophilus, L. bulgaricus, L. casei, L. fermentum, L. paracasei, L. plantarum, L. rhamnosus, and L. salivarius.

Acidophilus

Undoubtedly, acidophilus was the most popular name in probiotics from the early 1900s when Dr. Elie Metchnikoff identified lactobacilli as healthy flora for the well-being of the digestive tract and the longevity of life for the human race. From that time until the late 1960s, all probiotics were classified as acidophilus. However, the probiotic science and research have expanded tremendously with new discoveries and breakthroughs. Many new mutations and strains of bacteria have since then been identified to be as powerful as or stronger than the original acidophilus.

(Note: A warning that Lactobacillus acidophilus may cause serious infection was reported by the *Natural Health Remedies* newsletter by Jon Barron. People that have had injury or illnesses affecting their intestinal wall are at risk of infection. It can also cause infection of the heart lining in adults. Also, patients taking prescription drugs, such as prednisone, could be vulnerable to infections.[75]

There are many effective probiotic formulas available on the market today that do not contain acidophilus. (see page 81)

Some of the popular known species and their functions are listed below:

Lactobacillus acidophilus species exhibit an array of antimicrobial functions against many pathogenic activities. These include but are not limited to E. coli, salmonella, shigella, Helicobacter pylori, and candida.

Lactobacillus Rhamnosus

L. rhamnosus has excellent stability over a wide range of temperatures and pH levels; it relieves hypersensitivity reactions and intestinal inflammation in individuals with eczema and food allergies. It also has been found to strengthen the epidermal cells for a healthier and fungal-free skin.

L. rhamnosus strongly enhances the immune system through antagonizing and destroying foreign bacteria. It increases functions of antibody activity six to eight times above normal.[76]

L. rhamnosus produces more peptidases than any other Lactobacillus species. It favorably enhances innate and acquired immunity and causes outstanding colon epithelial cell adherence. It suppresses pathogenic Escherichia coli internalization. It supports gut microflora during antibiotic therapy.

---

[75] Jon Barron newsletter, July 2012.
[76] Barron's Report/The Probiotic Miracle, February 2011.

Lactobacillus Casei

L. casei has been found to have protective activity against pathogenic listeria bacteria.

Lactobacillus casei beneficially modulates innate immune responses. It increases the number of intestinal IgA-producing cells, antagonizes Helicobacter pylori, decreases cytokine secretion, inhibits E. coli adherence to intestinal cells, and decreases shigella-mediated inflammation.

Lactobacillus Plantarum

L. plantarum helps produce lactolin, a natural antibiotic, and synthesizes L. lysine.

L. plantarum is a highly beneficial transient bacteria generally lacking in people consuming a standard Western diet while universal in people consuming traditional plant-based diets. It supports intestinal barrier function, reduces translocation of gut bacteria, antagonizes C. difficile, and supports normal microflora in people with irritable bowel syndrome.

Many years ago, plantarum was a major part of people's diets (found in sauerkraut, etc.)

Lactobacillus Paracasei

L. paracasei exhibits super-high acid tolerance. It ferments inulin and phleins and produces high levels of lactic acid. It antagonizes C. difficile and staphylococcus aureus as well as other pathogens and contributes to a healthy vaginal microflora.

Lactobacillus Salivarius

L. Salivarius aids the intestinal tract in food digestion. It acts as a cleaning agent in the digestive tract. It eliminates fecal matter from the colon. It adheres to the wall of the intestines, therefore protecting the mucosal lining.

Bifidobacterium Species

The Bifidobacterium species are also lactic acid-producing bacteria like Lactobacillus. They are predominantly present in the large intestine.

Bifidobacterium Bifidum

Present in large numbers in a healthy colon. Populations are reduced in allergic infants and decline significantly with age. It supports gut microflora during antibiotic therapy and reduces positive testing for C. difficile toxins.

Bifidobacterium Longum

B. longum (biovar longum) has been found to eliminate nitrates from the intestinal tract.

B. longum ferments a broad spectrum of oligosaccharides. It is resistant to high bile and salt concentrations. It inhibits human neutrophil elastase, which may be important to innate immunity and attenuate harmful intestinal inflammation. It inhibits enterotoxigenic E. coli and favorably modulates inflammatory cytokine response to respiratory antigens. It improves inflammation in ulcerative colitis.

Bifidobacterium Lactis

Produces large amounts of antimicrobial fromate. It enhances leukocyte tumor-cell-killing properties and phagocytic activities. B. lactis significantly increases serum and mucosal IgA responses to cholera toxin and tetanus toxoid.

Streptococcus Thermophilus

Note: The particular streptococcus species is often known as highly pathogenic and not associated with health benefits. However, streptococcus thermophilus promotes healthy flora. It should not be confused with other streptococci species.

S. thermophilus generates lactase activity, facilitating the digestion of lactose in milk.

S. thermophilus is a transient species with a long history of use as a starter culture for yogurt and cheese. It is used for fermentation end products that inhibit pathogenic bacterial proliferation. It reduces DNA damage and premalignant lesion formation by protecting against carcinogens. It supports normal microflora and helps the gastrointestinal function in conditions ranging from rotavirus diarrhea in infants to remission in ulcerative colitis.

SAMPLING OF AN EFFECTIVE PROBIOTIC FORMULA OF MULTIPLE STRAINS

The following four probiotic strains are known to help relieve the rash and itching of skin fungus of the feet *and* yeast infections, but they do not stop there. These four strains are effective for many other health issues as well.

1. Bifidobacterium lactis—Scientific studies have proven this probiotic *enhances your immune system,* including increasing immunity among the elderly, resisting middle ear inflammation, lowering respiratory diseases, reducing colds and flu, curtailing allergies, increasing blood, Serum, controlling glucose, improving digestion, *lowering cholesterol,* and *fighting tumors.*

It is especially effective in *improving the skin* from attacking fungus.

2. Lactobacillus rhamnosus—Known to eliminate and *prevent the growth of harmful bacteria* in the intestines, this probiotic stimulates the production of antibodies and assists your body to combat invasive bacteria. It also has a high tolerance for the strong acids found in the digestive system, allowing maximum strength for *warding off disease and infection.*

3. Bifidobacterium bifidum—This is the *most ferocious good bacteria,* known to produce organic compounds including lactic acid, hydrogen peroxide, and acetic acid that halt reproduction of dangerous bacteria. Yeast (candida) is crowded out when hydrogen peroxide and acetic acid are present. *It synthesizes B-complex vitamins and absorbs calcium.*

Another study suggests it *helps prevent eczema*. Recent research says it controls diseases caused by allergic reactions.

4. Lactobacillus acidophilus—Means acid-loving milk-bacterium,[77] and it helps control the growth of oral and gastrointestinal infections. It also *facilitates digestion,* especially for those who are lactose-intolerant. It also *produces vitamin K* and helps control constipation and diarrhea.

A study published in the *Journal of the American College of Nutrition* reported it *reduces serum cholesterol,* potentially *lowering the risk for coronary heart disease.*

Because Lactobacillus acidophilus does not reside in your intestines or digestive tract, you must constantly replenish it daily for good health.

---

[77] Most Lactobacillus acidophilus produced today is milk-free and dairy-free and is certified as such from prominent independent laboratories. The original source was dairy, but the derivative is so far removed that biologically it has no trace of dairy whatsoever. It is usually declared safe for people who suffer from dairy intolerance.

PROBIOTIC ACHIEVEMENTS

A Synopsis

Probiotics have been protecting your digestive and immune systems for millennia. Modern-day probiotics, discovered in the early 1900s, are the precursor to our present-day production of man-made healthy microflora.

Many health benefits are conferred unto the digestive system and most organs of the human body, with probiotic consumption. The strengthening of the immune system and the aid in distribution of vitamins and minerals to the vital organs of the body are sufficient enough reasons that you should consume probiotics daily. The vast spectrum of healthy benefits realized in relieving other disorders are definitely an added bonus.

If your diet is vegetarian based and you consume healthy proteins and legumes, probiotics will assist your digestive tract to absorb the strength and energy into your system. If your diet is in the realm of the fast food industry, then probiotics are essential in protecting your intestinal tract from the invasion of multitudes of pathogens and carcinogenic bacteria.

Probiotic supplements are very special in that they have very few known adverse side effects. They can be taken alongside most medications without any adverse reactions. When they are taken for a specific malady or disorder, they provide additional strength and protection to a myriad of other areas in your body. They energize most vital parts of your body.

It is an amazing revelation that ten thousand times daily,[78] malfunctioning cells in your intestinal tract may become free radicals and might be carcinogenic. The healthy microflora in your gut, assisted with probiotic consumption, destroy them and never let them materialize.

We must be forever thankful to our Creator for His remarkable wisdom in which He created our body and its immune systems. He implemented a defense system that protects us more than ten thousand times every day from potentially damaging pathogens.

Ostensibly, probiotics could be the panacea for energizing and detoxifying your digestive tract and most organs of the human body.

Consumed daily, probiotics, together with a healthy diet and proper exercise, should help you enjoy a longer, healthier, and more energetic life.

Our journey into the world of probiotics has just begun!

---

[78]　See page 32 . . . .

PROBIOTIC TERMINOLOGY

Terms and Definitions

Antioxidant—A substance that protects key cell components by neutralizing the damaging effects of free radicals, natural by-products of cell metabolism that form when oxygen is metabolized or "burned" by the body.

Buffered—A process of adding alkaline substances to materials to counteract their acidity and neutralize the pH. The most common buffers used are magnesium, potassium, and calcium carbonates.

Candida—Yeast overgrowth in the intestinal tract that may cause vaginal infection.

Carcinogen—A substance that is directly involved in causing cancer.

Cellulitis—A bacterial infection affecting the deep layers of the outer skin. (Bacteria enter lacerated or cracked skin.) Cellulitis can attack any area of the body. It mostly appears on the legs.

CFU—A microbial colony-forming unit that is enumerated by direct count of viable, isolated bacterial colonies capable of growth on solid culture media.

cGMP—(Current Good Manufacturing Practices) Manufacturing guidelines recommended by the US Food and Drug Administration (FDA) to provide the best quality assurance for pharmaceutical and nutraceutical products.

Clostridium difficile—A bacterium that causes diarrhea and more serious intestinal conditions, such as Crohn's disease and IBS. It is a gram-positive, anaerobic, spore-forming bacillus that is responsible for the development of colitis.

Cytokines—The messengers of the immune system. Cytokines are substances, either proteins or glycoproteins, secreted by immune cells. In cancer therapy, cytokines are used to enhance immunity. Cytokines regulate the innate immune system: natural killer (NK) cells, macrophages, and neutrophil. They also regulate the adaptive immune system.

Dermatophytes—Types of fungi causing skin, hair, and nail infections known by the names ringworm and tinea. (When related to athlete's foot: tinea pedis. When related to jock itch: tinea cruris.)

Dysbiosis—An imbalance in the amounts of beneficial bacteria compared to yeast, harmful bacteria, viruses, or parasites in the digestive tract.

E. coli—These bacteria are medically known as enterotoxigenic Escherichia coli. E. coli food poisoning is a foodborne illness that is caused by the ingestion of E. coli bacteria. A symptom of E. coli poisoning is bloody diarrhea. Enterotoxigenic Escherichia coli, or ETEC (commonly referred to as E. coli), is an important cause of bacterial diarrhea illness. Infection with ETEC is the leading cause of traveler's disease. Enterotoxigenic Escherichia (ETEC) coli and shigella are two of the leading bacterial causes of diarrhea worldwide, together killing more than one million people every year.

Ecosystem—A biological environment of all organisms in a specific area of the body.

Epithelial cells—Cells from the skin that protect underlying tissue from mechanical injury, hence epithelial tissue. Epithelial cells help to protect or enclose organs; some produce mucus or other secretions.

Excipient—An inactive substance added to ingredients of medications or probiotics to enhance their absorbability into the various organs of the body.

Fromate—A probiotic compound used in fermentation of yogurt, etc.

Genus—A family of species (i.e., Lactobacillus or Bifidobacterium).

Gluten—A protein in grains, such as wheat, oats, rye, and barley. (Some people have allergic reactions to gluten.)

GRAS (Generally Recognized As Safe)—A term used by the Food and Drug Administration regarding food supplements on the market with a good and safe record.

Helicobacter pylori (H. pylori)—The bacteria responsible for most ulcers and many cases of stomach inflammation (chronic gastritis). The bacteria can weaken the protective coating of the stomach. It may bring on colitis or other digestive maladies.

Hypoallergenic—Products formulated to contain the fewest possible allergens so that they are not likely to cause an allergic reaction.

Hypochlorhydria—A condition of low hydrochloric acid levels in the stomach that is often the cause of digestive disorders.

Inulin—A type of dietary fiber extracted from chicory roots that supports the growth of healthy bacteria (prebiotics).

Lactose—The major sugar found in milk.

Leukocytes—There are two basic types of leukocytes: phagocytes and lymphocytes.

Lymphocytes—Cells that allow the body to remember and recognize their adversarial bacteria.

Mitochondria—The small organelles within a cell that control production of energy from food through ATP (adenosine triphosphate).

Neutrophil Elastase—It was hypothesized that neutrophil elastase released from activated neutrophils may play an important role in the pathogenesis of pulmonary fibrosis. For more information, visit: http://www.erj.ersjournals.com/cgi/content/abstract/11/1/120.

Neutrophils—A type of white blood cell or leukocyte that forms an early line of defense against bacterial infections.

Pathogens—Agents of infectious disease.

Peptidase—An enzyme that catalyzes the splitting of proteins into smaller peptide fractions and amino acids by a process known as proteolysis. Also called protease.

pH—Acid or alkaline measurement.

Phagocytes—Cells that chew up invading organisms.

Phagocytic Leukocytes—What is the role of phagocytic leukocytes? They are white blood cells that use phagocytosis to kill "foreign" objects in the blood stream. Neutrophils and monocytes are examples of active phagocytic leukocytes. For more information, visit: http://en.wikipedia.org/wiki/white_blood.

Phlebitis—Swelling of a vein caused by a blood clot, usually in the legs. Sometimes life threatening.

Prebiotics—Fructooligosaccharides (FOS) act as food for healthy flora in the digestive tract. Certain probiotic strains multiply up to one thousand times with added prebiotics.

Protease—Alternative name for peptidase.

Ringworm—The fungus causing athlete's foot fungus and some others.

Rotavirus—An infection that affects mostly children and is one of the most common causes of diarrhea. It is a viral infection of the digestive tract. It is the most common cause of severe diarrhea in infants and young children in the United States.

Species—An organism in a category capable of interbreeding (i.e., Lactobacillus, Bifidobacterium).

Stability Test—Test required by the Food and Drug Administration at the end of expiration date showing the full potency as stated on the bottle.

Strain—A subcategory of a species, in the same family of organisms (i.e., acidophilus, rhamnosus, bifidum).

Supernatant—Media source on which the probiotic culture was fermented.

T-cells (Lymphocytes)—White blood cells that help the body immune system recognize and memorize adverse bacteria and pathogens.

Xenobiotic—A substance that does not occur naturally and is foreign to the body, such as pesticide and industrial chemical.

INDEX

blood glucose levels, 63, 67
boron, 14
borscht, 1, 2, 3, 8
brain, 33, 46, 52, 57
bromelain (pineapple), 14
buffered, 105
Bulgaria, 7, 10
bulgaricus, 1, 6, 7, 96
buttermilk, 7, 8

C

cabbage, 3, 6, 7, 8, 76
cakes, 15
calcium, 14, 22, 66, 102
calcium carbonates, 105
calluses, 43–44
candida, 7, 42, 44, 45, 48, 73, 80, 92, 95, 97, 101, 105
candida albicans, 36, 42, 94
capsules, 68–69
caraway seeds, 2
caraway soup, 2–3
carbohydrates, 10, 15
carcinogenic activity defense, 94
carcinogens, 11, 22, 32, 56, 100, 104, 105
casein intolerance, 92
CAST (Council for Agricultural Science and Technology), xv
catalase, 14
cavities, 57–58
cecum, 16f
cellulitis, 45, 94, 105
centrifuge, 77, **78**
certification, 68
certified strains, 83–84
cervical skin erosions, 94, 95
CFUs (colony-forming units), 84–86, 105
cheese, 100

chemicals, impact on healthy flora of, 72
chocolate, dark, as prebiotic, 59
cholera toxin, 100
cholesterol, 60–62, 94, 101. *See also* HDL (high-density) cholesterol; LDL (low-density) cholesterol; serum cholesterol
chromium, 14
chronic gastritis, 51, 107
chyme, 24
circular muscle, 25f
citrus fruits, 6
cleanse/detoxification, 74–75
clostridium, 76
Clostridium difficile (C. difficile), 50–51, 53, 94, 98, 99, 106
cobalt, 14
colic, xvi, 53–54, 94
colitis, 50, 51, 71, 74, 94, 106, 107. *See also* ulcerative colitis
College of Medicine at Swansea University in Wales (UK), 48, 55
colon (large intestine), 15, 16f, 17, 18, 24, 26, 49, 51–52, 67, 69, 85, 99
colony-forming units (CFUs), 84–86, 105
common bile duct, 16f
constipation, 6, 18, 38, 51–52, 67, 88, 94, 102
The Consumer's Guide to Probiotics (Dash), 40, 60
controlled bacteria, 13
Cook, James, 5, 6
copolymer, 46
copper, 14
coronary heart disease, 102
coughing, 31
Council for Agricultural Science and Technology (CAST), xv

cradle cap, xvi, 37, 38, 48, 80, 94
Crohn's disease, 22, 49, 50, 94, 106
Culturelle Corp., 84
current good manufacturing practices (cGMP), 105
cystic acne, 47
cystitis (bladder inflammation), 23
cytokines, 98, 99, 106

D

dairy, cultivation of probiotics from, 13
dairy consumption, 56
dandruff, 7, 37, 44, 45–46, 48, 94
dark chocolate, as prebiotic, 59
Dash, S. K., 40, 52
DDS1, 83
defecation, 24
dermatologic eczema, 74
dermatophytes, 42, 44, 106
descending colon, 16*f*, 17
detoxification, 74, 94
diabetes, 61, 63–64, 94
diaper rash, 36, 48, 95
diarrhea, 6, 22, 49, 50, 52, 88, 95, 100, 102
diet, impact on healthy flora of, 72
dietary fiber, 66, 107
dieters, 56
digestion, 8, 11, 17, 18, 20, 22, 23, 24, 26, 27, 32, 58, 66, 72, 73, 99, 100, 101, 102
digestion timetable, 18
digestive cancers, 92
digestive enzymes, 8, 11, 13, 24, 53
digestive juices, 17,18
digestive system
    cleanse/detoxification of, 27, 74–75

enzymes as aiding, 15
    impact of fast food on, 10
digestive tract, impact of on immune system, 31–35
disease-causing bacteria, 22, 33
diverticulitis, 52
duodenum, 16*f*, 24
dysbiosis, 106

E

E. coli bacteria, 1, 2, 83, 95, 97, 98, 99, 106
eating habits, 10, 11, 49, 56, 57, 66, 91
ear sinus infections, 37–39
ecosystem, 15, 32, 106
eczema, 7, 37, 41, 42, 44, 80, 95, 97, 102. *See also* atopic eczema; dermatologic eczema
elimination process, 18
energy boosting, 93, 95, 103
enhanced dairy products, 15
enterobacteriaceae, 83
Enterotoxigenic Escherichia coli (ETEC), 106
enzymes, 11, 14, 17, 23, 25, 32, 56. *See also* digestive enzymes; human-manufactured enzymes
epidermal disorders, 73
epidermis, 7, 41, 42, 97
epithelial cells, 28, 106–107
epithelium, 20
esophagus, 15, 16*f*, 17, 20, 23
ETEC (Enterotoxigenic Escherichia coli), 106
European Journal of Clinical Nutrition, 54
The European Journal of Nutrition, 71
excipient, 28, 35, 107

refrigeration, 87, 89
regulated bowel movements, 73
rehydration therapy, 53
respiratory system, 31
rhamnosus, 55, 63, 76, 84, 96, 97, 101, 109
ringworm, 42, 43, 106, 109
rotavirus, 22, 100, 109
Royal Navy, 5–6

S

safety, of probiotics, 79–81
sales of probiotics (US), xvi
saliva, 23
salivary amylase, 14, 23
salivary glands, 14, 16*f*, 23
salmonella, 2, 76, 83, 95, 97
Sanders, Mary Ellen, xv
sauerkraut, 1, 3, 6, 8, 76, 98
scurvy, 5, 6
seaborne sicknesses, 5
sebum, 31
sedentary lifestyle, 91
selenium, 14
Seoul National University, 55
serosa, 25*f*, 26
serotonin, 33
serum cholesterol, 102
SFI (Symptom Frequency Index), 50
shampoo, ingredients that are toxic, 46
shelf life, 68, 69, 88–89
shigella, 2, 95, 97, 98
Shinshu Univrsity (Japan), 60
side effects, 81, 93
silicon, 14
simethicone, 54
single strains, 71–72
skin, 31, 41. *See also* epidermis
skin calluses, 43–44

skin maladies, 95
skin rash, 48
small intestine (ileum). *See* ileum (small intestine)
sneezing, 31
sodium, 14
soft drinks, 10
sour borscht, 1, 2, 3
sour milk, 7, 8
soy-free probiotics, 7
species, 109
spices, as prebiotic, 59
staining (excessive), 36
stability test, 109
staphylococcus aureus, 83, 98
starch digestion, 23
starches, 10
statin drugs, 61
Stilwell, R. H., 7
stomach, 14, 16*f*, 17, 18, 20, 23, 24
stomach inflammation, 51
stomach ulcers, 92
strains, 65, 69, 71–72, 77, 83–84, 85, 109
Streptococcus thermophilus, 100
submucosa, 25*f*
sugar, 15
sulphur, 14
super strains, 65, 69
supernatant, 65, 69, 109
supplements, 56
Swansea University in Wales (UK), 48, 55
symptoms relieved by probiotics, 94, 95
Symptom Frequency Index (SFI), 50
synbiotic effect, 71
synbiotics, 22, 66
synergistic effect, 71

T

tablets, 68, 69
Talmud, 2
Taylor, John, 29
t-cells (lymphocytes), 34, 109
tea, as prebiotic, 59
testing procedures, 82, 86
tetanus toxin, 100
thanking God for healthy digestive
  system, 25, 26, 34, 104
thrush, 36, 58, 95
tinea cruris, 42, 106
tinea pedis, 42, 43, 44, 106
tongue, 16f
toxins, 32, 33, 41, 47, 56, 88, 99,
  100
transverse colon, 16f, 17
triglycerides, 61, 62
type 2 diabetes, 63

U

UCLA, 47
ulcerative colitis, 22, 49, 50, 95,
  99, 100
ulcers, 51
unfriendly flora, 11
University of California at
  Berkeley, 53
University of Otago, Dunedin
  (NZ), 63
University of Pennsylvania, 34
University of Turku (Finland), 52
unsafe probiotics, 80
upper intestinal tract, 17
urinary tract infections (UTI), 23,
  36, 37, 73, 93, 95
urination, 64
uropathogenic bacteria, 36

V

vaginal infections, 95
vaginal microflora, 98
vaginitis, 95
vaginosis, 92
vanadium, 14
vascular system, 27
vegetable kingdom, 7
vegetables
  cultivation of probiotics from,
    13
  as prebiotic, 59
vegetarians, 72, 103
villi, 15, 17, 19f, 20, 21f, 22, 25f,
  26, 27, 57
virus contamination, 70, 82
viruses, 32, 95
vitamin A, 13
vitamin B1, 13
vitamin B2, 13
vitamin B3, 13
vitamin B5, 13
vitamin B6, 13
vitamin B12, 13
vitamin C (ascorbic acid), 6, 13
vitamin D, 13
vitamin E, 13
vitamin K, 13, 24, 102
vitamin therapy enhancements, 56
vitamins, 8, 11, 13, 15, 17, 25,
  27, 28, 32, 56, 72, 94. *See also*
  specific vitamins

W

washing of hands by doctors, 9
water-soluble vitamins, 13
weight loss, 57, 67
whole grains, as prebiotic, 59

women
  lower occurrence of athlete's
    foot fungus in, 44
  safety of probiotics for pregnant
    women, 63, 79, 80
The Wonder of Probiotics (Taylor),
  29
World Health Organization
  (WHO), 12, 52–53

X

xenobiotic, 109

Y

yeast, 83, 101
yeast fungus (candida), 36–37. *See
  also* candida
yeast infections, 23, 36, 37, 38, 39,
  44, 73, 80, 92, 93, 95
yeast overgrowth, 73
yogurt, 1, 8, 56, 100

Z

zinc, 14, 22, 66

www.ingramcontent.com/pod-product-compliance
Lightning Source LLC
Chambersburg PA
CBHW051424280526
45785CB00003B/1144